Obesity in the Dog and Cat

T0139099

Obesity in the Dog and Cat

Edited by
Martha G. Cline
Maryanne Murphy

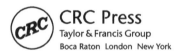

CRC Press
Taylor & Francis Group
Boca Raton London New York

CRC Press is an imprint of the
Taylor & Francis Group, an **informa** business

CRC Press
Taylor & Francis Group
6000 Broken Sound Parkway NW, Suite 300
Boca Raton, FL 33487-2742

© 2019 by Taylor & Francis Group, LLC
CRC Press is an imprint of Taylor & Francis Group, an Informa business

No claim to original U.S. Government works

Printed on acid-free paper

International Standard Book Number-13: 978-1-4987-4147-7 (Paperback)
978-0-367-20520-1 (Hardback)

Library of Congress Cataloging-in-Publication Data

Names: Cline, Martha G., editor.
Title: Obesity in the dog and cat / edited by Martha G. Cline, Maryanne Murphy.
Description: Boca Raton, Florida : CRC Press, [2019] | Includes bibliographical references and index.
Identifiers: LCCN 2019005133| ISBN 9781498741477 (paperback : alk. paper) | ISBN 9780367205201(hardback : alk. paper) | ISBN 9781315151625 (e-book : alk. paper).
Subjects: LCSH: Dogs--Diseases--Diet therapy. | Cats--Diseases--Diet therapy. | Obesity in animals.
Classification: LCC SF991 .O25 2019 | DDC 636.089/6398--dc23
LC record available at https://lccn.loc.gov/2019005133

**Visit the Taylor & Francis Web site at
http://www.taylorandfrancis.com**

**and the CRC Press Web site at
http://www.crcpress.com**

Dedication

We would like to dedicate this book to our spouses, B.J. and Cormac, for their infinite patience and support.

We would also like to dedicate this book to Colm, Clara, Ryder, Lennert, Jaxen, and Yona.

Contents

Preface

Veterinary medicine is facing a critical epidemic. Overweight and obese dogs and cats have a decreased quality of life, shortened life span, increased risk of other disease, and an overall increased cost of veterinary care. Veterinary professionals, from nurses to boarded specialists, should become fluent in the language of this epidemic.

General practice veterinarians and veterinary nurses are the target audience for this textbook . We began our careers after residency in a large private practice where specialists practiced veterinary medicine alongside general practitioners. Although many excellent resources regarding pet obesity exist, we saw a need to develop a comprehensive text to equip veterinary professionals on the first line. We also hope that those with a keen interest in veterinary nutrition will find this text an extensive resource of recent literature.

We would like to acknowledge the contributions of our authors. They manage pet obesity in clinical practice. They contribute to our body of knowledge surrounding pet obesity through research and publication. They educate future and current veterinary professionals on all aspects of obesity in veterinary medicine. The diverse experience and knowledge of these experts make this a beneficial resource for any veterinary professional.

Martha G. Cline
Maryanne Murphy

Editors

Dr. Martha G. Cline received her BS in biology from Lipscomb University in 2005 and her DVM from the University of Tennessee College of Veterinary Medicine in 2010. She subsequently completed a small animal rotating internship at Oradell Animal Hospital in New Jersey followed by a small animal clinical nutrition residency at the University of Tennessee. Dr. Cline became a Diplomate of the American College of Veterinary Nutrition in 2013 and then joined the staff at Red Bank Veterinary Hospital in Tinton Falls, NJ where she continues to practice clinical nutrition full time. Dr. Cline is the current President (2017–2019) of the American Academy of Veterinary Nutrition and has served on its Executive Board since 2013.

Dr. Maryanne Murphy received her dual BS in animal sciences and biological sciences from Rutgers University in 2004 and her DVM from Iowa State University in 2008, following which she completed a rotating general medicine and surgery internship at Fifth Avenue Veterinary Specialists in New York City and a clinical nutrition residency at the University of Tennessee. Dr. Murphy became a Diplomate of the American College of Veterinary Nutrition in 2013 and earned her PhD in Comparative and Experimental Medicine from the University of Tennessee in 2014. The focus of Dr. Murphy's dissertation research was energy metabolism and satiety in lean and obese dogs. She joined the staff of Red Bank Veterinary Hospital in Tinton Falls, NJ as a clinical nutritionist and then transitioned back to academia at the University of Tennessee in 2016 where she is a Clinical Assistant Professor of Nutrition. Dr. Murphy is currently Vice President of the American College of Veterinary Nutrition (ACVN).

Contributors

Charlotte Reinhard Bjørnvad, DVM, PhD, DECVCN
Section of Medicine, Oncology and Veterinary Clinical Pathology
Department of Veterinary Clinical Sciences
University of Copenhagen
Copenhagen, Denmark

Lene Elisabeth Buelund, DVM, PhD
Section of Veterinary Imaging
Department of Veterinary Clinical Sciences
University of Copenhagen
Copenhagen, Denmark

Martha G. Cline, DVM, DACVN
Red Bank Veterinary Hospital
Tinton Falls, New Jersey

Ashley Cox, BS, LVMT, VTS (Nutrition)
Department of Small Animal Clinical Sciences
College of Veterinary Medicine
University of Tennessee
Knoxville, Tennessee

Alexander J. German, BVSc, PhD, CertSAM, DECVIM-CA, SFHEA, FRCVS
Institute of Ageing & Chronic Disease and Institute of Veterinary Science
Faculty of Health & Life Sciences
University of Liverpool
Neston, United Kingdom

Kenneth J. Lambrecht, DVM
Bug Ventures Weight Management Systems
and
West Towne Veterinary Center
Madison, Wisconsin

Deborah E. Linder, DVM, DACVN
Department of Clinical Sciences
Cummings School of Veterinary Medicine
Tufts Institute for Human-Animal Interaction
Tufts University
North Grafton, Massachusetts

Lydia Love, DVM, DACVAA
Animal Emergency & Referral Associates
Fairfield, New Jersey

Andrew McGlinchey, DVM
VCA West Los Angeles
Los Angeles, California

Megan K. Mueller, MA, PhD
Department of Clinical Sciences
Cummings School of Veterinary Medicine
and
Jonathan M. Tisch College of Civic Life
Tufts University
North Grafton, Massachusetts

Maryanne Murphy, DVM, PhD, DACVN
Department of Small Animal Clinical
  Sciences
College of Veterinary Medicine
University of Tennessee
Knoxville, Tennessee

Elizabeth Orcutt, DVM, MS, DACVIM
Red Bank Veterinary Hospital
Tinton Falls, New Jersey

Valerie J. Parker, DVM, DACVIM, DACVN
Department of Veterinary Clinical
  Sciences
College of Veterinary Medicine
The Ohio State University
Columbus, Ohio

Angela Witzel Rollins, DVM, PhD, DACVN
Department of Small Animal Clinical
  Sciences
College of Veterinary Medicine
University of Tennessee
Knoxville, Tennessee

Megan Shepherd, DVM, PhD, DACVN
Department of Large Animal Clinical
  Sciences
Virginia-Maryland College of
  Veterinary Medicine
Blacksburg, Virginia

Justin Shmalberg, DVM, DACVN, DACVSMR
Department of Comparative,
  Diagnostic, and Population
  Medicine
College of Veterinary Medicine
University of Florida
Gainesville, Florida

Moran Tal, BSc, DVM, DVSc
Department of Clinical Studies
Ontario Veterinary College
University of Guelph
Guelph, Ontario, Canada

Adronie Verbrugghe, DVM, PhD, DECVCN
Department of Clinical Studies
Ontario Veterinary College
University of Guelph
Guelph, Ontario, Canada

Claudia Wong, DVM
Department of Clinical Studies
Ontario Veterinary College
University of Guelph
Guelph, Ontario, Canada

1

Epidemiology of small animal obesity

ADRONIE VERBRUGGHE

1.1 DEFINITION

Obesity results from a chronic positive energy balance, when caloric intake exceeds caloric needs, leading to excess body weight as body fat accumulates (1–3). Overweight pets are 10%–20% above ideal body weight; obese pets are more than 20% above ideal (4). Body composition studies note 25%–35% body fat is considered overweight and >35% obese (5,6). These obesity definitions should also include a component of disease, as excess body fat modifies bodily functions and contributes to disease processes (1–3).

1.2 PREVALENCE AND TIME TRENDS

Obesity is the number one nutrition problem in companion animals. The prevalence of canine obesity in industrialized countries is estimated at 11.2% to

59.4% (Table 1.1) (7–20). In cats, the prevalence rate ranges from 11.5% to 63.0% (Table 1.2) (10,21–32).

The presented data, however, has many limitations. The available studies spread a large time span and may not reflect the situation today. Moreover, studies have been conducted in a limited number of veterinary practices or were performed in very specific pet populations, using a variety of techniques to estimate body condition leading to various definitions of overweight/obesity. Also the person assessing the pet's body condition varies among studies.

Differences between countries and time trends are therefore difficult to investigate. A relatively constant distribution of body condition was noted in a cat population over a 4-year timespan (22,23). Also cat households surveyed in the same city in 1993 and 2007 did not show a difference of obesity prevalence (26,31).

1.3 RISK FACTORS

Obesity is a multifactorial condition. Many risk factors affect energy intake and energy utilization, creating a positive energy balance (1,2). Veterinarians believe that only 3% of obese cases were attributed to animal-specific factors, while 97% was caused by human-specific factors such as dietary factors, physical activity, owner attitudes, and household characteristics (Figure 1.1) (33).

1.3.1 Animal-specific factors

1.3.1.1 GENETICS AND BREED

Genetic factors of obesity are illustrated by breed predisposition. Still, the obesity frequency in specific dog breeds depends on the breed prevalence in the region of study. Overall, basset hounds, beagles, cairn terriers, cocker spaniels, dachshunds, golden retrievers, Labrador retrievers, pugs, and Shetland sheepdogs are among the predisposed breeds (8,9,13,14,18–20). Selection for a specific purpose or physical condition may be the reason. For some dog breeds the breeding standard seems to be overweight (19,20). Moreover, body composition varies among breeds (34), influencing energy expenditure (35). Contrary, crossbred cats are at higher risk to be overweight (22,24,27,28). Nonetheless, British shorthair, Persian, and Norwegian Forest cat have higher body condition scores among purebreds (32,36).

1.3.1.2 AGE

The obesity prevalence increases with age (8,11–13,18,22,31), due to decreasing energy requirements especially as physical activity declines and age-related body composition changes cause the basal metabolic rate to drop (37,38). Harper described a 20% decrease in dogs, yet observed constant energy requirements throughout adult life in cats (37). Bermingham et al. could however not confirm a decline of energy requirements in aging dogs (39), yet did find an age-related reduction of energy expenditure in cats (40). Epidemiological studies report the highest prevalence of obesity in the middle-aged years for both dogs (12,14,18) and

Table 1.1 Prevalence of obesity in various canine populations in various countries over 55-year time period (from 1960 to 2015)

Authors	Year	Country	Population	Sample size	Evaluation method	Prevalence rate
Krook et al. (7)	1960	Sweden	Canine necropsies	10,993	Pathologist Presence of pathologic adiposity	Obese: 11.2%
Mason (8)	1970	UK	One veterinary practice	1000	Attending veterinarian 3-point scale: thin, normal or obese, fat covering thorax	Obese: 28.0%
Edney and Smith (9)	1986	UK	11 veterinary practices, ranging from veterinary schools to private practices	8268	Attending veterinarians 5-point scale: thin, lean, optimum, obese, gross	Obese/gross: 24.3%
Lund et al. (10)	1999	USA	52 veterinary practices	86,772	Attending veterinarians 5-point scale: fat covering ribs and tail base and abdominal contour.	BCS ≥4/5: 28.3%
Robertson (11)	2003	Australia	2326 households, telephone survey	657	Owners 3-point scale: underweight, correct weight, overweight/obese	Overweight/ obese: 25.2%
McGreevy et al. (12)	2005	Australia	209 veterinary practices	2661	Attending veterinarians: 5-point scale: Hill's weight guide chart for dogs and cats showing silhouettes	BCS ≥4/5: 1.1%
Colliard et al. (13)	2006	France	Vaccination service of veterinary school	616	Attending veterinarian 5-point scale, adapted from Laflamme (5)	BCS ≥4/5: 38.8%

(Continued)

Table 1.1 (*Continued*) Prevalence of obesity in various canine populations in various countries over 55-year time period (from 1960 to 2015)

Authors	Year	Country	Population	Sample size	Evaluation method	Prevalence rate
Lund (14)	2006	USA	52 veterinary practices	21,754	Attending veterinarians 5-point scale: fat covering ribs and tail base and abdominal contour	BCS ≥4/5: 34.1%
Courcier et al. (15)	2010	UK	One charitable and 4 private first-opinion veterinary practices	696	Attending veterinarians or student veterinarians Morphometric technique adapted from a 7-point scale S.H.A.P.E.™ score (74)	S.H.A.P.E.™ ≥5/7: 59.4%
Sallander et al. (16)	2010	Sweden	Owners of pure-bred, dogs registered with large animal-insurance company, telephone survey	461	Owners 5-point scale: very lean, lean, normal, obese and very obese, using pictures after Laflamme (5) and previously validated (75,76)	Obese/very obese: 16.0%
Heuberger and Wakshlag (17)	2011	USA	Dog owners recruited using word of mouth and advertisement, mail survey	61	Owners 5-point scale: underweight, slightly underweight, ideal weight, slightly overweight, obese	Slightly overweight/obese: 21.3%
Mao et al. (18)	2013	China	14 veterinary practices	2391	Attending veterinarians: 5-point scale (4,5)	BCS ≥4/5: 44.4%
Corbee (19)	2013	Netherlands	One dog show	1379	Board Certified Veterinary Nutritionist™ 9-point scale (5)	BCS ≥6/9: 19.8%
Such and German (20)	2015	UK	Photographs of dogs that appeared at a dog show	960	Veterinarian with experience in assessing BCS from photographs 9-point scale and previously validated (77)	BCS ≥6/9: 26.0%

Abbreviations: BCS: body condition score; S.H.A.P.E.™: Size, Health And Physical Evaluation.

Table 1.2 Prevalence of obesity in the feline population in various countries, and time trends over 23 years (from 1992 to 2015)

Authors	Year	Country	Population	Sample size	Evaluation method	Prevalence rate
Sloth (21)	1992	Denmark	One veterinary practice	233	Attending veterinarian 4-point scale: underweight, normal weight, overweight, obese weight	Overweight/obese: 40.0%
Scarlett et al. (22)	1994	USA	31 veterinary practices	2091	Attending veterinarians 6-point scale: cachectic, lean, optimal-lean, optimal, heavy, and obese using silhouettes	Heavy/obese: 25.0%
Donoghue and Scarlett (23)	1998	USA	27 veterinary practices, information from previously studied cats (22)	1654	Attending veterinarians 6-point scale (22)	Heavy/obese: 24.5%
Lund et al. (10)	1999	USA	52 veterinary practices	42,774	Attending veterinarians 5-point scale: fat covering ribs and tail base and abdominal contour, adapted from Scarlett et al. (22)	BCS ≥4/5: 27.5%
Robertson (24)	1999	Australia	2195 households, telephone survey	644	Owner 3-point scale: underweight, correct weight, overweight (obese)	Overweight/obese: 18.9%
Russell et al. (25)	2000	UK	Households, door-to-door visit	136	Experienced assessor 17-point scale adapted from Laflamme (6)	Overweight/obese: 52%

(Continued)

Table 1.2 (Continued) Prevalence of obesity in the feline population in various countries, and time trends over 23 years (from 1992 to 2015)

Authors	Year	Country	Population	Sample size	Evaluation method	Prevalence rate
Allan et al. (26)	2000	New Zealand	492 households, door-to-door survey	182	Experienced assessor 3-point scale: normal weight, overweight, obese, assessing inguinal, abdominal and subcutaneous fat	Overweight/obese: 25.8%
Lund et al. (27)	2005	USA	52 veterinary practices	8159	Attending veterinarians 5-point scale: fat covering ribs and abdominal contour	BCS $\geq$4/5: 35.1%
Colliard et al. (28)	2009	France	Vaccination service at veterinary school	385	Attending veterinarian 5-point scale adapted from Laflamme (6)	BCS $\geq$4/5: 26.8%
Courcier et al. (29)	2010	UK	One charity first-opinion veterinary practice	118	Student veterinarian 5-point scale adapted from Laflamme (6)	BCS $\geq$4/5: 39.0%
Courcier et al. (30)	2012	UK	47 charity first-opinion veterinary practices	3219	Attending veterinarians 5-point scale	BCS $\geq$4/5: 11.5%
Cave et al. (31)	2012	New Zealand	1045 households, door-to-door survey, similar to Allen et al. (26)	200	Two independent experienced assessors 9-point scale (6)	BCS $\geq$7/9[a]: 27.4% BCS $\geq$6/9: 63.0%
Corbee (32)	2014	Netherlands	Two cat shows	268	Board Certified Veterinary Nutritionist™ 9-point scale (6)	BCS $\geq$6/9: 45.5%

Abbreviation: BCS: body condition score.

[a] The validated 9-point scale (6) can be compressed into the non-validated 5-point scale, where 1/9 is equivalent to 1/5; 2–3/9 = 2/5, 4–6/9 = 3/5, 7–8/9 = 4/5, and 9/9 = 5/5 (31).

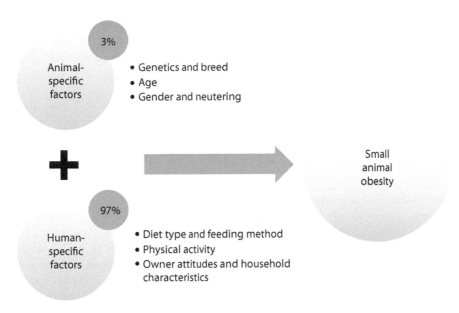

Figure 1.1 Risk factors of small animal obesity, including animal-specific and human-specific factors. Percentages according to Bland et al. (33).

cats (22,24,27,28,30). The obesity frequency declines after about 10 years of age (12,22), as overweight animals may have a shorter lifespan because of detrimental health effects (41).

1.3.1.3 GENDER AND NEUTERING

Epidemiological data show an overrepresentation of overweight female dogs (7,8,12,13,15,16,18), which may be related to differences in body composition and energy requirements. Male dogs have more lean tissue compared to females (42), suggesting lower energy requirements in females, predisposing them to weight gain. Still, a recent meta-analysis could not confirm that gender affects energy requirements of dogs (39). In cats, lower energy requirements have been confirmed in females compared to males (43), while males are unexpectedly more at risk to become overweight (22,24,27,28,30,36).

A key link exists between neutering and obesity (9,11,13,14,18,21,22,24,27–30, 32,36). Neutered dogs are 2.8 times (11) and neutered cats 3.6 times more likely to be overweight than their intact counterparts (30). A higher frequency of obesity was also reported in dogs neutered between 5.5 and 12 months of age compared to before 5.5 months (44). The latter, however, could not be confirmed in cats (45). This link occurs due to removal of sex hormones. A reduction of estrogen-induced appetite suppression may occur in females (46). When fed *ad libitum*, female Beagles consumed more food postneutering and their body weight increased more compared to intact controls (46). Similar effects were noted in neutered cats when compared to intact controls or to before surgery (47–49). At the same time, substantial food restriction is necessary to maintain ideal body weight postneutering in queens (49,50) and bitches (51). Also resting energy expenditure is 30% lower after gonadectomy in cats of both genders (52,53). At last, neutering also leads to a reduction in spontaneous activity, because of decreased roaming and sexual behavior, especially among males (54,55).

1.3.2 Human-specific factors

1.3.2.1 DIET TYPE AND FEEDING METHOD

Highly palatable, energy dense foods put pets at risk for weight gain, especially when fed free-choice. Dietary fat is the most concentrated and most efficiently stored energy source (3). In dogs (56) and cats (57,58), high-fat, low-carbohydrate diets resulted in more body fat and weight gain compared to low-fat, high-carbohydrate diets. Nonetheless, all macronutrients (fat, protein and carbohydrates) are stored as body fat and will all lead to weight gain when fed in excess (3). Conversely, inclusion of dietary fiber, water or air can decrease energy density. In dogs, a positive association between high dietary fiber content and normal body condition has been reported (17).

Most studies found no influence of commercial diet types on the obesity prevalence (9,11,15,24,26,29,31). Though, some reported higher risk in cats consuming "premium" dry foods and/or therapeutic diets (22,27,28), probably because of higher energy density compared to most economy type diets (22,27). Also, owners tend to feed dry food *ad libitum* (23). Despite an increased proportion of owners feeding dry food, Australian researchers noted no association with dry food feeding in 1993 (26) and 2007 (31), and no increase of obesity occurred over this period (31). Moreover, epidemiological studies cannot determine whether the findings associated with therapeutic diets are cause or effect. It is also noteworthy that confounding may have occurred as low-energy therapeutic diets are prescribed for weight loss (27,28). Likewise, dogs and cats fed homemade food, table scraps, and/or treats are more inclined to obesity (8,11,14–18,59,60).

Free-choice or *ad libitum* feeding contributes to excess energy intake, while dividing the daily portion into multiple meals may increase energy loss from thermogenesis (61) and physical activity (62). Research disagrees on the effect of *ad libitum* feeding and feeding frequency, which can often not be teased apart. Depending on the study, dogs are at higher risk to become obese when fed once a day (11), when receiving several meals (18), or when fed either one or three-plus portions (59). In cats, *ad libitum* feeding or feeding frequency has been shown to be a risk factor by some (25,48,60) but not by others (22,24,26,28,31), and one study found the opposite, that is, cats fed twice daily were more likely to be obese than cats fed *ad libitum* (29). Food items may be given only once or twice per day, but may be available all day (24). Also division of the appropriate daily portion into small meals and providing excess energy by feeding free-choice food throughout the day should not be confused.

Overall, overfeeding is more important. Determining the daily portion based on package instructions may lead to excess energy intake, as recommendations are based on ranges and averages of energy requirements. Owners overestimate their pet's activity level (63) and underestimate their pet's body condition

(13,26,29,31,64–66), increasing the likelihood to overfeed. Seventy percent of cat owners feed until their cat stops eating, while only 8% follow package instructions and only 4% ask their veterinarian (29). Besides, most pet owners do not weigh the food with a gram scale but rather use a measuring cup. This is quick and convenient, but also imprecise and inaccurate, contributing to the obesity epidemic (67).

1.3.2.2 PHYSICAL ACTIVITY

Lack of exercise has also been identified as a major risk factor (11,15,18,21,22,24,26,59); especially as low levels of physical activity reduce energy expenditure (68). Most studies attributed this to the type of habitat. Obese pets tend to live indoors and may have restricted opportunities for exercise (11,21,22,24,26). Still, two feline studies could not associate activity with obesity, probably because of differences in confinement between countries and because the owner's assessment of activity is biased (25,31). Habitat may, however, not be the best indicator. Dogs with garden access as an exercise regime, rather than walks, are more likely to be obese (59). And dogs residing in apartments are walked more frequently than dogs living in a detached house (69). Overall, the risk of canine obesity decreases with each hour of weekly exercise (11,15), yet the intensity of exercise (walking versus running) did not affect obesity (11). Unfortunately, most pet owners overestimated their dog's activity level as they consider their dogs moderately to very active (63). Also less active pets tend to have less active owners (70).

1.3.2.3 OWNER ATTITUDES AND HOUSEHOLD CHARACTERISTICS

In general, obese pets are overhumanized by their owners and have a potential role as substitute for human companionship. For example, obese dogs sleep more often in the owner's bed and owners of obese pets talk more to their dog and cat (60,71). These pets are no longer treated as typical companion animals, ignoring needs such as exercise, play, work, protection, and environmental enrichment (60,71). The pet's health and nutritional needs are also ignored (60,71). Behavior signals are often misread, causing overfeeding as owners assume the pet is hungry when it is not and food is frequently used as reward (71). Owners of overweight dogs also have less interest in balanced dog nutrition (71,72) and will especially pay attention to low price and special offers rather than quality of ingredients and nutritional composition when buying dog food (71,72). This is partly due to a lower income among these owners (15,71), but also results from their own health and eating habits (71). Owners of obese dogs often suffer from obesity as well (8,13,17,71,73). They may engage less in exercise and pay less attention to a healthy diet. Owners who ate low-calorie diets had nonobese dogs (17). In cats however, no correlation could be found between the degree of overweight of cats and the body mass index of their owners (60,73). Studies also report a higher risk of obesity for dogs kept by middle-aged or elderly people than when kept by adults under 40 years of age (8,13,15). This was attributed to lack of exercise (8), yet owner age did not affect the amount of exercise a dog received (15). Moreover, older people own the oldest dogs (13). Likewise cat owner's age was not a real risk factor, as the owner's age also confounded the cat's age (28). Additionally, one would think that children may give too many treats or overfill the food bowl; yet living with one child was reported to lower the obesity risk in cats (28). Also households with only one dog (11) or only one or two cats (22,24) showed a higher risk, while the presence of dogs reduced the risk of cats to become obese (26).

Owners underestimating their pet's body condition (8,13,15,26,28,29,31,60,65,66) is another reason to overfeed and has been identified to be a major factor in feline obesity (26,28,29,31). For example, owners who consider their normal weight cats to be underweight may be encouraged to feed more (28) and if owners don't perceive their pet to be overweight, owners will not be motivated to reduce the pet's energy intake (31). Likewise, if informed by their veterinarian that their dog is overweight, owners may be either reluctant to accept this judgment or may not think this is an important concern (65).

1.4 CONCLUSION

Numerous risk factors including animal-specific factors and human-specific factors are involved in pet obesity, making for a disease that is often hard to tackle. Risk factors should be identified by a thorough nutritional assessment in every pet at every veterinary health exam to prevent weight gain or to achieve weight loss. Animal-specific factors can be targeted in individualized calculations of daily energy requirements. However, of utmost importance is owner education and elimination of human-specific factors, such as dietary factors, physical activity, owner attitudes, and household characteristics, which contribute the most to the obesity epidemic.

REFERENCES

1. German AJ. The growing problem of obesity in dogs and cats. *The Journal of Nutrition* 2006;136(7 Suppl):1940S–1946S.
2. Laflamme DP. Understanding and managing obesity in dogs and cats. *Veterinary Clinics of North America: Small Animal Practice* 2006;36(6):1283–1295, vii.
3. Laflamme DP. Companion animals symposium: Obesity in dogs and cats: What is wrong with being fat? *Journal of Animal Science* 2012;90(5):1653–1662.
4. Burkholder WJ. Use of body condition scores in clinical assessment of the provision of optimal nutrition. *Journal of the American Veterinary Medical Association* 2000;217(5):650–654.
5. Laflamme D. Development and validation of a body condition score system for dogs. *Canine Practice* 1997;22(4):10–15.
6. Laflamme D. Development and validation of a body condition score system for cats: A clinical tool. *Feline Practice* 1997;25(5–6):13–18.
7. Krook L, Larsson S, Rooney JR. The interrelationship of diabetes mellitus, obesity, and pyometra in the dog. *American Journal of Veterinary Research* 1960;21:120–127.

8. Mason E. Obesity in pet dogs. *The Veterinary Record* 1970;86(21): 612–616.
9. Edney AT, Smith PM. Study of obesity in dogs visiting veterinary practices in the United Kingdom. *The Veterinary Record* 1986;118(14):391–396.
10. Lund EM, Armstrong PJ, Kirk CA, Kolar LM, Klausner JS. Health status and population characteristics of dogs and cats examined at private veterinary practices in the United States. *Journal of the American Veterinary Medical Association* 1999;214(9):1336–1341.
11. Robertson ID. The association of exercise, diet and other factors with owner-perceived obesity in privately owned dogs from metropolitan Perth, WA. *Preventive Veterinary Medicine* 2003;58(1–2):75–83.
12. McGreevy PD, Thomson PC, Pride C, Fawcett A, Grassi T, Jones B. Prevalence of obesity in dogs examined by Australian veterinary practices and the risk factors involved. *The Veterinary Record* 2005;156(22):695–702.
13. Colliard L, Ancel J, Benet JJ, Paragon BM, Blanchard G. Risk factors for obesity in dogs in France. *Journal of Nutrition* 2006;136(7):1951S–1954S.
14. Lund EM, Armstrong PJ, Kirk CA, Klausner JS. Prevalence and risk factors for obesity in adult dogs from private US veterinary practices. *International Journal of Applied Research in Veterinary Medicine* 2006;4(2):177–186.
15. Courcier EA, Thomson RM, Mellor DJ, Yam PS. An epidemiological study of environmental factors associated with canine obesity. *Journal of Small Animal Practice* 2010;51(7):362–367.
16. Sallander M, Hagberg M, Hedhammar A, Rundgren M, Lindberg JE. Energy-intake and activity risk factors for owner-perceived obesity in a defined population of Swedish dogs. *Preventive Veterinary Medicine* 2010;96(1–2):132–141.
17. Heuberger R, Wakshlag J. The relationship of feeding patterns and obesity in dogs. *Journal of Animal Physiology and Animal Nutrition* 2011;95(1):98–105.
18. Mao J, Xia Z, Chen J, Yu J. Prevalence and risk factors for canine obesity surveyed in veterinary practices in Beijing, China. *Preventive Veterinary Medicine* 2013;112(3–4):438–442.
19. Corbee RJ. Obesity in show dogs. *Journal of Animal Physiology and Animal Nutrition* 2013;97(5):904–910.
20. Such ZR, German AJ. Best in show but not best shape: A photographic assessment of show dog body condition. *The Veterinary Record* 2015;177(5):125.
21. Sloth C. Practical management of obesity in dogs and cats. *Journal of Small Animal Practice* 1992;33(4):178–182.
22. Scarlett JM, Donoghue S, Saidla J, Wills J. Overweight cats: Prevalence and risk-factors. *International Journal of Obesity* 1994;18:S22–SS8.
23. Donoghue S, Scarlett JM. Diet and feline obesity. *Journal of Nutrition* 1998;128(12 Suppl):2776S–2778S.

24. Robertson ID. The influence of diet and other factors on owner-perceived obesity in privately owned cats from metropolitan Perth, Western Australia. *Preventive Veterinary Medicine* 1999;40(2):75–85.
25. Russell K, Sabin R, Holt S, Bradley R, Harper EJ. Influence of feeding regimen on body condition in the cat. *The Journal of Small Animal Practice* 2000;41(1):12–17.
26. Allan FJ, Pfeiffer DU, Jones BR, Esslemont DHB, Wiseman MS. A cross-sectional study of risk factors for obesity in cats in New Zealand. *Preventive Veterinary Medicine* 2000;46(3):183–196.
27. Lund EM, Armstrong PJ, Kirk CA, Klausner JS. Prevalence and risk factors for obesity in adult cats from private US veterinary practices. *International Journal of Applied Research in Veterinary Medicine* 2005;3(2):88–96.
28. Colliard L, Paragon BM, Lemuet B, Bénet JJ, Blanchard G. Prevalence and risk factors of obesity in an urban population of healthy cats. *Journal of Feline Medicine and Surgery* 2009;11(2):135–140.
29. Courcier EA, O'Higgins R, Mellor DJ, Yam PS. Prevalence and risk factors for feline obesity in a first opinion practice in Glasgow, Scotland. *Journal of Feline Medicine and Surgery* 2010;12(10):746–753.
30. Courcier EA, Mellor DJ, Pendlebury E, Evans C, Yam PS. An investigation into the epidemiology of feline obesity in Great Britain: Results of a cross-sectional study of 47 companion animal practises. *The Veterinary Record* 2012;171(22):560.
31. Cave NJ, Allan FJ, Schokkenbroek SL, Metekohy CA, Pfeiffer DU. A cross-sectional study to compare changes in the prevalence and risk factors for feline obesity between 1993 and 2007 in New Zealand. *Preventive Veterinary Medicine* 2012;107(1–2):121–533.
32. Corbee RJ. Obesity in show cats. *Journal of Animal Physiology and Animal Nutrition* 2014;98(6):1075–1080.
33. Bland IM, Guthrie-Jones A, Taylor RD, Hill J. Dog obesity: Veterinary practices' and owners' opinions on cause and management. *Preventive Veterinary Medicine* 2010;94(3–4):310–315.
34. Jeusette I, Greco D, Aquino F, Detilleux J, Peterson M, Romano V et al. Effect of breed on body composition and comparison between various methods to estimate body composition in dogs. *Research in Veterinary Science* 2010;88(2):227–232.
35. Arch JR, Hislop D, Wang SJ, Speakman JR. Some mathematical and technical issues in the measurement and interpretation of open-circuit indirect calorimetry in small animals. *International Journal of Obesity* 2006;30(9):1322–1331.
36. Kienzle E, Moik K. A pilot study of the body weight of pure-bred client-owned adult cats. *British Journal of Nutrition* 2011;106(1 Suppl):S113–S115.
37. Harper EJ. Changing perspectives on aging and energy requirements: Aging and energy intakes in humans, dogs and cats. *Journal of Nutrition* 1998;128(12 Suppl):2623S–2626S.

38. Harper EJ. Changing perspectives on aging and energy requirements: Aging, body weight and body composition in humans, dogs and cats. *Journal of Nutrition* 1998;128(12 Suppl):2627S–2631S.
39. Bermingham EN, Thomas DG, Cave NJ, Morris PJ, Butterwick RF, German AJ. Energy requirements of adult dogs: A meta-analysis. *PLOS ONE* 2014;9(10):e109681.
40. Bermingham EN, Weidgraaf K, Hekman M, Roy NC, Tavendale MH, Thomas DG. Seasonal and age effects on energy requirements in domestic short-hair cats (*Felis catus*) in a temperate environment. *Journal of Animal Physiology and Animal Nutrition* 2013;97(3):522–530.
41. Kealy RD, Lawler DF, Ballam JM, Mantz SL, Biery DN, Greeley EH et al. Effects of diet restriction on life span and age-related changes in dogs. *Journal of the American Veterinary Medical Association* 2002;220(9):1315–1320.
42. Lauten SD, Cox NR, Brawner WR, Baker HJ. Use of dual energy x-ray absorptiometry for noninvasive body composition measurements in clinically normal dogs. *American Journal of Veterinary Research* 2001;62(8):1295–1301.
43. Bermingham EN, Thomas DG, Morris PJ, Hawthorne AJ. Energy requirements of adult cats. *British Journal of Nutrition* 2010;103(8):1083–1093.
44. Spain CV, Scarlett JM, Houpt KA. Long-term risks and benefits of early-age gonadectomy in dogs. *Journal of the American Veterinary Medicine Association* 2004;224(3):380–387.
45. Spain CV, Scarlett JM, Houpt KA. Long-term risks and benefits of early-age gonadectomy in cats. *Journal of the American Veterinary Medical Association* 2004;224(3):372–379.
46. Houpt KA, Coren B, Hintz HF, Hilderbrant JE. Effect of sex and reproductive status on sucrose preference, food intake, and body weight of dogs. *Journal of the American Veterinary Medical Association* 1979;174(10):1083–1085.
47. Fettman MJ, Stanton CA, Banks LL, Hamar DW, Johnson DE, Hegstad RL et al. Effects of neutering on bodyweight, metabolic rate and glucose tolerance of domestic cats. *Research in Veterinary Science* 1997;62(2):131–136.
48. Harper EJ, Stack DM, Watson TDG, Moxham G. Effects of feeding regimens on bodyweight, composition and condition score in cats following ovariohysterectomy. *Journal of Small Animal Practice* 2001;42(9):433–438.
49. Belsito KR, Vester BM, Keel T, Graves TK, Swanson KS. Impact of ovariohysterectomy and food intake on body composition, physical activity, and adipose gene expression in cats. *Journal of Animal Science* 2009;87(2):594–602.
50. Flynn MF, Hardie EM, Armstrong PJ. Effect of ovariohysterectomy on maintenance energy requirement in cats. *Journal of the American Veterinary Medical Association* 1996;209(9):1572–1581.

51. Jeusette I, Detilleux J, Cuvelier C, Istasse L, Diez M. Ad libitum feeding following ovariectomy in female Beagle dogs: Effect on maintenance energy requirement and on blood metabolites. *Journal of Animal Physiology and Animal Nutrition* 2004;88(3–4):117–121.
52. Root MV, Johnston SD, Olson PN. Effect of prepuberal and postpuberal gonadectomy on heat production measured by indirect calorimetry in male and female domestic cats. *American Journal of Veterinary Research* 1996;57(3):371–374.
53. Martin L, Siliart B, Dumon H, Backus R, Biourge V, Nguyen P. Leptin, body fat content and energy expenditure in intact and gonadectomized adult cats: A preliminary study. *Journal of Animal Physiology and Animal Nutrition* 2001;85(7–8):195–199.
54. Hart BL, Barrett RE. Effects of castration on fighting, roaming, and urine spraying in adult male cats. *Journal of the American Veterinary Medical Association* 1973;163(3):290–292.
55. Hopkins SG, Schubert TA, Hart BL. Castration of adult male dogs: Effects on roaming, aggression, urine marking, and mounting. *Journal of the American Veterinary Medical Association* 1976;168(12):1108–1110.
56. Romsos DR, Belo PS, Bennink MR, Bergen WG, Leveille GA. Effects of dietary carbohydrate, fat and protein on growth, body composition and blood metabolite levels in the dog. *Journal of Nutrition* 1976;106(10):1452–1464.
57. Backus RC, Cave NJ, Keisler DH. Gonadectomy and high dietary fat but not high dietary carbohydrate induce gains in body weight and fat of domestic cats. *British Journal of Nutrition* 2007;98(3):641–650.
58. Nguyen PG, Dumon HJ, Siliart BS, Martin LJ, Sergheraert R, Biourge VC. Effects of dietary fat and energy on body weight and composition after gonadectomy in cats. *American Journal of Veterinary Research* 2004;65(12):1708–1713.
59. Bland IM, Guthrie-Jones A, Taylor RD, Hill J. Dog obesity: Owner attitudes and behaviour. *Preventive Veterinary Medicine* 2009;92(4): 333–340.
60. Kienzle E, Bergler R. Human-animal relationship of owners of normal and overweight cats. *Journal of Nutrition* 2006;136(7 Suppl):1947S–1950S.
61. LeBlanc J, Diamond P. Effect of meal size and frequency on postprandial thermogenesis in dogs. *American Journal of Physiology* 1986;250(2 Pt 1): E144–E147.
62. Deng P, Iwazaki E, Suchy SA, Pallotto MR, Swanson KS. Effects of feeding frequency and dietary water content on voluntary physical activity in healthy adult cats. *Journal of Animal Science* 2014;92(3): 1271–1277.
63. Slater MR, Robinson LE, Zoran DL, Wallace KA, Scarlett JM. Diet and exercise patterns in pet dogs. *Journal of the American Veterinary Medical Association* 1995;207(2):186–190.
64. Courcier EA, Mellor DJ, Thomson RM, Yam PS. A cross sectional study of the prevalence and risk factors for owner misperception of canine body

shape in first opinion practice in Glasgow. *Preventive Veterinary Medicine* 2011;102(1):66–74.

65. White GA, Hobson-West P, Cobb K, Craigon J, Hammond R, Millar KM. Canine obesity: Is there a difference between veterinarian and owner perception? *Journal of Small Animal Practice* 2011;52(12):622–626.

66. Eastland-Jones RC, German AJ, Holden SL, Biourge V, Pickavance LC. Owner misperception of canine body condition persists despite use of a body condition score chart. *Journal of Nutritional Science* 2014;3:e45.

67. German AJ, Holden SL, Mason SL, Bryner C, Bouldoires C, Morris PJ et al. Imprecision when using measuring cups to weigh out extruded dry kibbled food. *Journal of Animal Physiology and Animal Nutrition* 2011;95(3):368–73.

68. Larsson C, Junghans P, Tauson AH. Evaluation of the oral ^{13}C-bicarbonate tracer technique for the estimation of CO_2 production and energy expenditure in dogs during rest and physical activity. *Isotopes in Environmental and Health Studies* 2010;46(4):432–443.

69. Degeling C, Burton L, McCormack GR. An investigation of the association between socio-demographic factors, dog-exercise requirements, and the amount of walking dogs receive. *Canadian Journal of Veterinary Research* 2012;76(3):235–240.

70. Chan CB, Spierenburg M, Ihle SL, Tudor-Locke C. Use of pedometers to measure physical activity in dogs. *Journal of the American Veterinary Medical Association* 2005;226(12):2010–2015.

71. Kienzle E, Bergler R, Mandernach A. A comparison of the feeding behavior and the human–animal relationship in owners of normal and obese dogs. *Journal of Nutrition* 1998;128(12 Suppl):2779S–2782S.

72. Suarez L, Peña C, Carretón E, Juste MC, Bautista-Castaño I, Montoya-Alonso JA. Preferences of owners of overweight dogs when buying commercial pet food. *Journal of Animal Physiology and Animal Nutrition* 2012;96(4):655–659.

73. Nijland ML, Stam F, Seidell JC. Overweight in dogs, but not in cats, is related to overweight in their owners. *Public Health Nutrition* 2010;13(1):102–106.

74. German AJ, Holden SL, Moxham GL, Holmes KL, Hackett RM, Rawlings JM. A simple, reliable tool for owners to assess the body condition of their dog or cat. *Journal of Nutrition* 2006;136(7 Suppl):2031S–2033S.

75. Sallander M, Hedhammar A, Rundgren M, Lindberg JE. Demographic data of a population of insured Swedish dogs measured in a questionnaire study. *Acta Veterinaria Scandinavica* 2001;42(1):71–80.

76. Sallander MH, Hedhammar A, Rundgren M, Lindberg JE. Repeatability and validity of a combined mail and telephone questionnaire on demographics, diet, exercise and health status in an insured-dog population. *Preventive Veterinary Medicine* 2001;50(1–2):35–51.

77. Gant PH, Holden SL, Biourge V, Morris PJ, German AJ. Can body composition in dogs be estimated from photographs? *Journal of Veterinary Internal Medicine* 2013;27:742.

2

Pathophysiology of obesity: Metabolic effects and inflammation mediators

ANGELA WITZEL ROLLINS AND MEGAN SHEPHERD

2.1 BALANCING ENERGY EXPENDITURE AND INTAKE

In its most simplistic state, obesity is caused by an imbalance between energy intake and energy expenditure. However, the factors leading to increased calorie consumption or decreased energy use are complicated and multifactorial. So why has obesity reached epidemic proportions in both humans and companion animals? Studies evaluating twins and family associations find genetics account for approximately 65% of the variance in obesity and body mass index (BMI) in people (1–6). It also appears that most of the remaining variance in BMI results from differences in individuals rather than shared environmental effects (1). In dogs, certain breeds (see Chapter 1) have higher rates of obesity than others (7). While genetics certainly play a role regarding individual variation of adiposity, the dramatic increase in obesity rates over the past 50 years cannot be fully attributed to genetic changes alone. The prevalence of obesity in U.S. adults has more than doubled since the early 1960s, increasing from 13.4% to 35.7% (8,9). While most experts agree our modern societal changes in food availability and sedentary behaviors have combined with a susceptible genetic background to create the perfect scenario for weight gain, several theories to further clarify this relationship exist.

2.1.1 Evolutionary theories of obesity

One of the earliest theories explaining modern obesity was the thrifty gene hypothesis (10). This is the idea that natural selection placed pressure on thinner individuals during famines. Those with slower metabolisms and a greater ability to retain fat mass were more likely to survive the harsh environments of the past. In addition, higher levels of body fat would better sustain fertility during times of famine. One potential flaw to this theory is that if natural selection even slightly favored a genetic mutation toward obesity over the course of human evolution, we would expect approximately 99% of people to currently be affected (11).

An alternative theory is that lean individuals had an evolutionary advantage in that they would be faster to avoid predators (11). As societies developed and there were more stable food supplies with less predation, a wider population of individuals and body types could survive. This relaxation of selection resulted in genetic drift that allowed obese phenotypes, or "drifty genes" (11).

It is well known that certain human races and ethnic groups have higher rates of obesity compared to others. A more recent hypothesis for the predisposition of some groups toward weight gain involves the presence of brown adipose tissue (BAT) and uncoupling protein 1 (UCP1) gene. Both BAT and UCP1 mediate the release of energy in the form of heat. Infants and children have high concentrations of BAT, which is important for survival and thermogenesis. In addition, humans and animals living in colder climates tend to have more BAT and higher expression of UCP1. The release of energy as heat also results in a higher metabolic rate. Humans evolving in warmer climates may have slower metabolisms related to lower concentrations and expression of BAT and UPC1. This "thermogenic" theory of obesity evolution could account for higher obesity rates found in American Indian, black, and Hispanic populations (12,13).

Most of the evolutionary theories of human obesity center on a genetic predisposition for weight gain when exposed to new dietary or activity patterns. The rise in canine and feline obesity in recent years could also be the result of these environmental pattern changes. Most companion animals have easy access to highly palatable, energy-dense diets. In addition, more cats and dogs are kept confined indoors with few opportunities for exercise compared to their ancestors. A popular theory emerging for cats is the idea that they evolved as strict carnivores and the high carbohydrate concentrations in commercial cat foods are contributing to a feline obesity epidemic. While there is evidence that a lower carbohydrate diet (35 g/1000 kcal vs. 76 g/1000 kcal) better regulates blood glucose concentrations in diabetic cats (14) and can reduce postprandial insulin and glucose concentrations in healthy cats (15,16), there is currently no evidence that dietary carbohydrate content directly impacts the risk or development of obesity. On the contrary, studies have found cats fed a high fat (63 g/1000 kcal; 54 g/1000 kcal CHO) or high protein (124 g/1000 kcal; 62 g/1000 kcal CHO) versus a high carbohydrate (126–137 g/1000 kcal; 58–80 g/1000 kcal protein; 29–32 g/1000 kcal fat) diet gain more fat mass and consume more calories (15,17). Whether long-term feeding of high carbohydrate diets contributes to the development of diabetes in cats remains unclear. While more research is needed to elucidate the role of carbohydrates in the development of obesity, there are some environmental factors such as indoor housing and *ad libitum* feeding patterns that appear more frequently in obese versus lean cats; however, this is not consistently identified (18–20). For example, the impact of feeding a mostly dry diet on obesity is mixed with one study showing a significant correlation while another found no association (19,21; see Chapter 1). Several studies have also failed to show a connection between feeding patterns or outdoor activity and obesity (22–24).

Theories regarding evolutionary pressure combined with changes in modern society are not the only hypotheses regarding the development of obesity. Other theoretical factors currently being investigated to account for the dramatic rise in obesity include infectious agents such as viruses and bacteria, gut microflora alterations (see Section 2.3), endocrine disruption from environmental contaminants, and psychosocial stress (25). Additionally, the ways in which appetite and food intake are regulated via central, peripheral, and hedonic controls must be considered.

2.1.2 Regulation of appetite and food intake

2.1.2.1 CENTRAL REGULATION OF APPETITE

While the regulation of appetite and food intake within the central nervous system is a complex process, the main control center is the arcuate nucleus of the hypothalamus. Within this area of the brain are neurons that express proopiomelanocortin (POMC) and cocaine- and amphetamine-regulated transcript (CART). These signaling molecules reduce appetite and increase energy expenditure and are often described as *anorexigenic*. There are also neurons that express agouti-related protein (AgRP) and neuropeptide Y (NPY), and increase appetite while decreasing energy expenditure. These neurons are referred to as *orexigenic* (Figure 2.1). Hormonal signals from peripheral tissues like the stomach and adipose tissue stimulate the hypothalamus to excite or inhibit these neurons to affect appetite. Neurons within the arcuate nucleus also communicate with

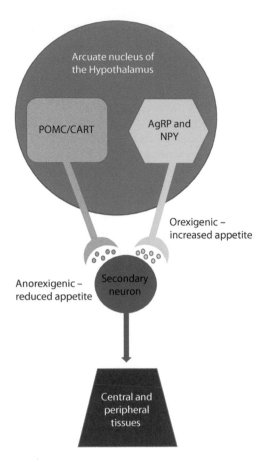

Figure 2.1 Central appetite control occurs within the arcuate nucleus of the hypothalamus. Neurons expressing proopiomelanocortin (POMC) and cocaine- and amphetamine-regulated transcript (CART) neuropeptides reduce appetite and increase energy expenditure and are termed anorexigenic. Neurons expressing agouti-related protein (AgRP) and neuropeptide Y (NPY) increase appetite while decreasing energy expenditure and are termed orexigenic.

other anorexigenic and orexigenic neurons in other areas of the hypothalamus to regulate food intake (26).

2.1.2.2 PERIPHERAL REGULATION OF APPETITE

To determine when the body needs more or less food, the brain and hypothalamus must rely on other organs and tissues to communicate both immediate and long-term energy needs. For example, stretch receptors in the stomach can prevent overdistension by signaling the brain to end a meal, and adipose tissue sends hormonal signals to tell the brain when fat stores increase or decrease. One of the best studied adipose hormones is leptin. As an individual gains excess body fat, more leptin is released from adipocytes (fat cells). Leptin travels to the hypothalamus where it stimulates the anorexigenic neurons to reduce food intake and increase energy expenditure. On the other hand, if an individual is losing weight and fat stores decrease, lower concentrations of leptin and reduced release of POMC and CART increase appetite and slow the metabolic rate. Thus, leptin works to keep a more or less constant state of adiposity and is sometimes referred to as an *adipostat*, similar to a thermostat, for fat mass (27). In addition to signaling long-term energy stores, leptin can also signal acute reductions in energy intake. For example, a study of healthy men undergoing 2–3 days of fasting showed dramatic reductions in serum leptin concentrations (28). While leptin attempts to prevent excess weight gain through appetite control, obese individuals tend to have higher concentrations of leptin and can become resistant to leptin's effects. Thus, similar to insulin resistance, leptin resistance results in ineffectual hormone action despite high circulating levels (29). There is some indirect evidence that leptin resistance may also occur in dogs and cats. Many studies have demonstrated higher circulating levels of leptin with increased fat mass in both dogs and cats, but no studies have correlated leptin with voluntary food intake (30–36).

In addition to adipose tissue, the gut is critical for signaling food intake to the brain. As mentioned earlier, stretch receptors in the stomach and intestine signal distention from meal ingestion and travel via the vagus nerve to stimulate the central appetite controls. There are also numerous gut peptides that are released in the presence of energy-containing nutrients, with small dietary proteins and amino acids being the primary triggers. With the exception of the hormone ghrelin, which is released from the stomach and stimulates hunger and food-seeking behaviors, all known gut peptides suppress appetite. Cholecystokinin (CCK), peptide YY (PYY), and glucagon-like peptide-1 (GLP-1) are three of the best characterized gut peptides regulating appetite, and they indirectly stimulate the hypothalamic region via stimulation of the vagus nerve and brain stem (37).

2.1.2.3 HEDONIC (PLEASURE) CONTROL OF APPETITE

While the hypothalamus and other areas of the brain rely on physiologic cues to control appetite, current research in humans also implicates higher brain centers related to reward, attention, emotions, and other cognitive control systems in the regulation of food intake (26). These higher centers are in direct communication with the hypothalamus and can often override physiologic satiety signals.

Eating gives pleasure and stimulates reward centers of the brain. However, the role of food reward can become altered in obese states. One theory states that obese individuals have lower availability of dopamine 2 receptors in the striatum of the brain. As a result, they require highly rewarding (high fat or high calorie) foods to feel content. However, some evidence suggests the exposure to high fat or high calorie foods itself is to blame for lower dopamine 2 receptor levels. This theory of hyporesponsiveness to food reward is often equated to a food addiction, similar to a drug addiction. A second theory linking food reward to obesity claims exposure to high-reward foods leads to a hyperresponse in the reward center and causes individuals to desire greater quantities of food. While both theories demonstrate a role of the reward systems in dysregulated appetite and obesity, more controlled studies are needed (26).

In humans, it has been well demonstrated that emotions can modify appetite. For example, anxiety and depression are common comorbidities of obesity. Anger and joy increase appetite and create poor food choices when compared to sadness and fear (38). While it may be difficult to extrapolate these finding to companion animals, we know that dogs and cats have complex emotional feelings, and energy intake is likely influenced to some extent by their emotional state.

2.1.3 Mechanisms of energy expenditure and metabolic control

As mentioned in the beginning of the chapter, obesity is an imbalance between energy consumed and energy expended. Maintenance energy requirement (MER) is the amount of energy needed each day to maintain a steady body weight and is made up of the following sections (39):

- Basal metabolism
- Thermogenesis
- Physical activity
- Anabolic development—growth, pregnancy, lactation

Animals oxidize proteins, fats, and carbohydrates in a stepwise manner that frees energy in small, useable amounts through the creation of CO_2, H_2O, and energy. This process is known as *catabolism*. Within the body, high-energy phosphate bonds are stored in the form of fats, proteins, and carbohydrates, and the creation of these energy storage forms is termed *anabolism* (40).

The basal metabolic rate (BMR) makes up a large portion of energy burned and is defined as the amount of energy utilized after a 12-hour fast while lying down, awake, in a thermoneutral environment. It is the energy needed to maintain blood circulation, respiration, and metabolic activities of cells. The term *resting energy requirement* (RER) is often used by veterinary nutritionists to describe an energy state similar to BMR. BMR and RER are often estimated across species using the Kleiber interspecies formula: Body weight$^{0.75}_{(kg)} \times 70$ (41). The amount of fat-free mass (lean tissue like organs and muscle) are the best predictors of BMR and RER since fat mass accounts for very little of basal energy (39). Therefore, the preceding equation is best utilized with an animal's ideal weight rather than using overweight mass (42).

Thermogenesis affects basal metabolism by expending energy during the digestion and processing of food, termed *thermic effect of food* (TEF), and by maintaining a stable core body temperature despite variations in the outside environment. Basal metabolism and thermogenesis are influenced by various factors. The thyroid gland and its hormones play a large role in energy expenditure of metabolically active tissues such as the liver, brown adipose tissue, skeletal muscle, and the heart. Thyroid hormones also promote the generation of energy for thermogenesis by reducing thermodynamic efficiency. This leads to increased heat production and body temperature. When the ambient temperature falls outside of an animal's thermoneutral zone, most mammals employ heat-saving and generating mechanisms like shivering, vasoconstriction, and piloerection. For long-term thermogenesis, mammals will also utilize brown adipose tissue, which contains a mitochondrial protein in the cells that generates heat. BAT thermogenesis is modulated by the hypothalamus with norepinephrine as the key neurotransmitter and thyroid hormones in a supporting role (43). When consuming a meal with proteins, fats, and carbohydrates, about 10% of the calories ingested will go toward the TEF (39). The amount of energy utilized during physical activity is the most variable component of the MER. There exists a wide range of MER in dogs, 94 to $250 \, \text{kcal} \times \text{BW}_{(kg)}^{0.75}$, and most of this variation is due to differences in daily activity and exercise (44).

2.2 INFLAMMATORY EFFECTS OF OBESITY

2.2.1 Endocrine functions of adipose tissue

A variety of endocrine, paracrine, and autocrine signals are released from cells within adipose tissues. These signals are referred to as adipokines. The term *adipokine* is generally used to describe any protein released by adipose tissue regardless of whether it is released by adipocytes or nonfat cells (45). Although many adipokines have been discovered, the function and physiologic relevance of most have not been identified. A few adipokines have been intensively studied and appear to positively or negatively impact insulin sensitivity. While the metabolic role of most adipokines is complex and incompletely understood, leptin, adiponectin, and tumor necrosis factor alpha (TNF-α) are some of the most intensely studied adipokines.

Leptin was the first adipokine identified and its main function is to regulate body fat mass through appetite control and increased energy metabolism (see subsection on peripheral control of appetite). Although leptin's primary physiologic role is to regulate body fat storage, it also affects the immune, cardiovascular, and reproductive systems (46,47). Leptin may also enhance insulin signaling to improve intracellular glucose uptake and decrease the accumulation of lipid in peripheral tissues (48). Genetically mutant rodents that can't produce leptin, referred to as *ob/ob*, develop obesity, insulin resistance, and diabetes (49,50). On the other hand, leptin can have pro-inflammatory and mitogenic (cancer-causing) properties because it stimulates production of various pro-inflammatory cytokines (see discussion of inflammation in Section 2.2.2) (51).

Adiponectin is the most abundantly secreted adipokine in circulation (52). Although adipocytes are responsible for secreting adiponectin, hormone levels become paradoxically lower with increased fat mass (53). The reason behind this unusual relationship is not clear. It is speculated that increased levels of other adipokines, such as TNF-α, may suppress adiponectin expression. Adiponectin exerts a myriad of metabolic affects. Perhaps the most influential role of adiponectin is as an insulin sensitizer. Adiponectin is closely associated with insulin sensitivity, independent of body fat mass (54–56). Prospective and longitudinal studies in human beings demonstrate that lower adiponectin levels are closely associated with insulin resistance and future development of diabetes (57–59). Higher levels of adiponectin are also strongly associated with reduced risk of type 2 diabetes in healthy adult human beings (60). Numerous clinical and epidemiological studies associate low levels of adiponectin with chronic inflammatory states such as obesity, insulin-resistance, type 2 diabetes, hypertension, cardiovascular disease, and liver disease (61,62).

Adiponectin research in companion animals has yielded mixed results. While most studies demonstrate an inverse relationship with body fat in cats (34,63,65–67), other studies have shown poor correlation (30,68,69). Differences in measurement techniques and study design may account for some of the discrepancies. In addition, most studies in cats measure total adiponectin rather than the more active high molecular weight form, and this may reduce the ability to find relationships. To date, only two studies have evaluated the multimeric forms of adiponectin to body fat mass in cats and both found the high molecular weight fraction of adiponectin was more closely associated with body fat percentage than total adiponectin (30,68). Research regarding adiponectin in dogs tells a similar story with some studies showing a negative correlation with body fat (35,71,72,74) and others finding no consistent relationship (36,75–77).

TNF-α is an inflammatory cytokine expressed by a variety of cells including macrophages, mast cells, neuronal cells, fibroblasts, and adipocytes. The connection between TNF-α, obesity, and insulin resistance is unclear. Since TNF-α can be secreted by both differentiated and undifferentiated adipocytes, it was thought that the increased levels of TNF-α found in obesity were primarily due to adipocyte secretion; however, cells within the stromovascular fraction of adipose tissue, including macrophages, produce significantly more TNF-α than adipocytes (79–81). TNF-α secretion from adipose tissue has key species differences. In human beings, most adipose TNF-α exerts local paracrine and autocrine actions (82,83). In mice and dogs, more TNF-α is released into systemic circulation (75,84). The circulation patterns of TNF-α derived from adipose tissue are not well understood in cats, but mRNA expression within fat is increased with obesity (86). One of the primary actions of adipose TNF-α, regardless of the species, is induction of localized insulin resistance. TNF-α downregulates genes responsible for insulin-mediated glucose uptake into cells (87–89). In addition to inhibiting glucose entry into cells, TNF-α decreases uptake of free fatty acids (FFA) into adipocytes and promotes lipolysis and release of FFA into circulation (80,82,90). As a result, FFA levels increase in circulation and negatively affect insulin sensitivity in peripheral tissues. In addition to directly influencing insulin sensitivity of adipose tissue, TNF-α can alter secretion of other adipokines involved in glucose metabolism. In particular, TNF-α inversely correlates with adiponectin and may alter its gene expression (80,82,91,92). In summary, TNF-α secreted from adipose tissue plays an important role in glucose and lipid metabolism at both the local and systemic level, and is a key component to inflammation associated with obesity.

2.2.2 Obesity and inflammation

It is well known that obese individuals tend to live in a state of chronic, low-grade inflammation directly related to excess adipose tissue. This inflammatory state is thought to contribute to the development of cancer and other chronic diseases in humans. Increased adiposity is estimated to cause approximately 20%–35% of many types of human cancers (93,94). While the mechanisms behind obesity and cancer development are tumor specific, many cancer types may develop secondary to inflammatory conditions (93). The two methods by which this inflammatory state arises can be simplified into local inflammation at the level of the adipocytes themselves and systemic release of inflammatory mediators from adipose tissue.

2.2.2.1 LOCAL INFLAMMATION

Adipocytes develop from multipotent stromal stem cells (MSCs). Increased adiposity must come from either hypertrophied adipocytes that are larger and contain more triglyceride or from hyperplasia with increased numbers of adipocytes. Except under extreme circumstances, adult humans are relatively stable in the number of adipocytes they possess. However, children can easily undergo adipocyte hyperplasia and increase their number of fat cells for life (95,96).

One well-known side effect of obesity is inflammation. It is thought that hypoxia within adipose tissue is a main factor for inducing inflammation. Obese humans and rodents have been shown to have reduced adipose tissue blood flow. In addition, oxygen can only diffuse through about 120 μm of tissue and adipocytes can be as large as 150 μm (97). Obese mice also appear to have reduced angiogenesis and increased vasoconstriction (97). Chronic inflammatory states result in overproduction of reactive oxygen species (ROS) and systemic oxidative stress. High levels of oxidative stress are thought to be a key link between obesity, vascular abnormalities, and the elevated risk of atherosclerosis and cardiovascular disease in humans (98).

2.2.2.2 SYSTEMIC INFLAMMATION

As mentioned earlier, two hormones released from adipose tissue play key roles in inflammation throughout the body. Concentrations of the anti-inflammatory hormone adiponectin decrease with increased fat mass while the pro-inflammatory hormone leptin increases in concentrations. Leptin stimulates production of inflammatory cytokines like IL-6, IL-12, IL-1, and TNFα by the innate immune system. It also stimulates production of nitric oxide, cyclooxygenase 2 (COX2), nitric oxide, and reactive oxygen species (51). In addition to alterations in adipokine expression, obesity enhances activity of the renin–angiotensin system, which can increase intracellular ROS, mitochondrial dysfunction, and DNA damage (99).

2.3 ROLE OF THE MICROBIOME IN OBESITY

2.3.1 Gut microbiota and obesity

The gastrointestinal tract microbial population (gut microbiota) has profound effects on host health, and an association between the gut microbiota and obesity has been established (100,101). The majority of investigations of the obese gut microbiota have been carried out in humans and rodents. Generally, the gut microbiota of obese individuals is characterized by a reduced diversity (102–106). The taxa-level alterations, such as the abundance of *Firmicutes* phylum members in the gut or feces of obese versus lean individuals of the same species, varies between studies. For the dog, signatures of obese versus lean lack consistency across the few studies published (107,108). The variation across studies could be due to variation across study cohorts, such as client-owned versus colony dogs or the effect of environment on gut microbes (109). Furthermore, the variation could also be explained by the lack of consensus in methods for evaluating the complex gut, or often fecal, microbiota (110). Employing gut microbes in disease management is challenging because the membership of the gut microbiota does not directly reflect function as there are conserved functions across broad bacterial taxonomic groups. Proposed mechanisms by which gut microbes may influence obesity include altered digestion and dietary energy extraction, enhanced lipogenesis and fat storage, and appetite regulation (100,105,111–114); these mechanisms have not yet been studied in the dog or cat.

2.3.2 Utility of the gut microbiota in obesity management

2.3.2.1 DIETARY STRATEGIES

Diet influences the canine gut microbiota (115) and gut microbiota of other species. This should be no surprise since microbes are efficient and quickly adjust to changes in available substrate. Some of the various anti-obesity dietary interventions (i.e., enhancing fiber, altering fat, or enhancing polyphenols) are associated with parallel alterations in the gut microbiota or prevention of dysbiosis (116,117). These studies link diet, gut microbiota, and obesity; however, the link between gut microbiota and obesity isn't fully elucidated. Furthermore, other investigations of similar dietary interventions show the influence of diet to be independent of changes in the gut microbiota (118,119). Currently, there does not seem to be a practical means to engage the diet gut microbiota dynamic in the management of canine obesity (120). However, research on the role of diet in modulating obesity through the gut microbiome is still being developed.

2.3.2.2 NONDIETARY STRATEGIES

Probiotics are typically live microbial species that provide health benefits. Probiotics have been suggested as a strategy for treating obesity through gut microbiota modulation and altering metabolism (121). Comparing the beneficial effect of probiotics across studies is challenging due to variation in manufacturing, strain inclusion, number of strains and form (powder, chew, etc.). The more popular bacterial genera in canine probiotic supplements include *Lactobacillus*, *Bifidobacterium*, and *Enterococcus* species (121–123). These popular probiotic bacteria have not yet been shown to help prevent obesity (124,125) and may be more helpful in promoting weight gain (126). Probiotics are generally considered safe for dogs; however, probiotics are not free of risks and have been associated with bacteremia and fungemia in compromised human neonates and elderly patients (127,128).

Antibiotics alter the gut microbiota of dogs (129) as well, but due to concerns with antimicrobial resistance in dogs (130,131), this nondietary strategy may be considered unethical. Transfaunation, transfer of gut or fecal (repoopulation) contents, is an older method for transferring healthy gut microbes from a healthy host to a sick host (132) that has seen a recent resurgence in use (85,133,134). Transfaunation for obesity management does not look promising to date as there is more evidence that transfaunation promotes weight gain (73,78,100,119) than weight loss (64). Establishment of the gut microbiota begins before birth (70) and generally is resistant to change in adulthood. Therefore, future strategies addressing the role of the dam and neonatal management on gut microbes may provide the most promise.

2.4 CONCLUSION

Although it is easy to describe obesity as the result of energy intake exceeding energy expenditure, it is clear that such a relationship is complex and affected by a myriad of factors. The genetic makeup and environment of our patients play enormous roles in the development of excess adipose tissue. For example, the middle-aged, hypothyroid Labrador retriever will likely have to consume fewer calories per kilogram to maintain a lean body weight compared to a young-adult Weimaraner. We also now realize that obesity has systemic effects on the entire body, and the pro-inflammatory state produced by excess adipose tissue contributes to chronic illnesses such as cancer and diabetes mellitus. By better understanding the causes and consequences of obesity, veterinarians will be better able communicate with pet owners and devise effective weight loss plans.

REFERENCES

1. Speakman JR, Westerterp KR. A mathematical model of weight loss under total starvation: Evidence against the thrifty-gene hypothesis. *Disease Models & Mechanisms* 2013;6(1):236–251.
2. Allison DB, Kaprio J, Korkeila M, Koskenvuo M, Neale MC, Hayakawa K. The heritability of body mass index among an international sample of monozygotic twins reared apart. *International Journal of Obesity and Related Metabolic Disorders: Journal of the International Association for the Study of Obesity* 1996;20(6):501–506.
3. Segal NL, Allison DB. Twins and virtual twins: Bases of relative body weight revisited. *International Journal of Obesity and Related Metabolic Disorders: Journal of the International Association for the Study of Obesity* 2002;26(4):437–441.
4. Luke A, Guo X, Adeyemo AA et al. Heritability of obesity-related traits among Nigerians, Jamaicans and US black people. *International Journal of Obesity and Related Metabolic Disorders: Journal of the International Association for the Study of Obesity* 2001;25(7):1034–1041.

5. Wu X, Cooper RS, Borecki I et al. A combined analysis of genomewide linkage scans for body mass index from the National Heart, Lung, and Blood Institute Family Blood Pressure Program. *American Journal of Human Genetics* 2002;70(5):1247–1256.

6. Zhu X, Cooper RS, Luke A et al. A genome-wide scan for obesity in African-Americans. *Diabetes* 2002;51(2):541–544.

7. Lund EM, Armstrong PJ, Kirk CA, Klausner JS. Prevalence and risk factors for obesity in adult dogs from private US veterinary practices. *International Journal of Applied Research in Veterinary Medicine* 2006;4:177–186.

8. Ogden CL, Carroll MD. *Prevalence of overweight, obesity, and extreme obesity among adults: United States, trends 1960–1962 through 2007–2008. NCHS Health E-Stat.* Hyattsville, MD: National Center for Health Statistics; 2010. Available online: http://www.cdc.gov/NCHS/data/hestat/obesity_adult_07_08/obesity_adult_07_08.pdf.

9. Flegal KM, Carroll MD, Kit BK, Ogden CL. Prevalence of obesity and trends in the distribution of body mass index among US adults, 1999–2010. *Journal of the American Medical Association* 2012;307(5):491–497. Available online: http://jama.jamanetwork.com/article.aspx?articleid=1104933.

10. Neel J. Diabetes mellitus a "thrifty" genotype rendered detrimental by "progress"? *American Journal of Human Genetics* 1962;14:352–353.

11. Speakman JR. Thrifty genes for obesity, an attractive but flawed idea, and an alternative perspective: The 'drifty gene' hypothesis. *International Journal of Obesity* 2008;32(11):1611–1617.

12. Albuquerque D, Stice E, Rodriguez-Lopez R, Manco L, Nobrega C. Current review of genetics of human obesity: From molecular mechanisms to an evolutionary perspective. *Molecular Genetics and Genomics* 2015;290(4):1191–1221.

13. Sellayah D, Cagampang FR, Cox RD. On the evolutionary origins of obesity: A new hypothesis. *Endocrinology* 2014;155(5):1573–1588.

14. Bennett N, Greco DS, Peterson ME, Kirk C, Mathes M, Fettman MJ. Comparison of a low carbohydrate-low fiber diet and a moderate carbohydrate-high fiber diet in the management of feline diabetes mellitus. *Journal of Feline Medicine & Surgery* 2006;8(2):73–84.

15. Coradini M, Rand JS, Morton JM, Rawlings JM. Effects of two commercially available feline diets on glucose and insulin concentrations, insulin sensitivity and energetic efficiency of weight gain. *The British Journal of Nutrition* 2011;106(Suppl 1):S64–S77.

16. Farrow HA, Rand JS, Morton JM, O'Leary CA, Sunvold GD. Effect of dietary carbohydrate, fat, and protein on postprandial glycemia and energy intake in cats. *Journal of Veterinary Internal Medicine* 2013;27(5):1121–1135.

17. Gooding MA, Atkinson JL, Duncan IJH, Niel L, Shoveller AK. Dietary fat and carbohydrate have different effects on body weight, energy expenditure, glucose homeostasis and behaviour in adult cats fed to energy requirement. *Journal of Nutritional Science* 2015;4:e2.

18. Russell K, Sabin R, Holt S, Bradley R, Harper EJ. Influence of feeding regimen on body condition in the cat. *Journal of Small Animal Practice* 2000;41(1):12–17.
19. Harper EJ, Stack DM, Watson TD, Moxham G. Effects of feeding regimens on bodyweight, composition and condition score in cats following ovariohysterectomy. *The Journal of Small Animal Practice* 2001;42(9):433–438.
20. Kienzle E, Bergler R. Human-animal relationship of owners of normal and overweight cats. *The Journal of Nutrition* 2006;136(7 Suppl):1947S–1950S.
21. Rowe E, Browne W, Casey R, Gruffydd-Jones T, Murray J. Risk factors identified for owner-reported feline obesity at around one year of age: Dry diet and indoor lifestyle. *Preventive Veterinary Medicine* 2015;121(3–4):273–281.
22. Cave NJ, Allan FJ, Schokkenbroek SL, Metekohy CA, Pfeiffer DU. A cross-sectional study to compare changes in the prevalence and risk factors for feline obesity between 1993 and 2007 in New Zealand. *Preventive Veterinary Medicine* 2012;107(1–2):121–133.
23. Scarlett JM, Donoghue S, Saidla, Wills J. Overweight cats: Prevalence and risk factors. *International Journal Obesity Related Metabolic Disorders* 1994;S22–S28.
24. Allan FJ, Pfeiffer DU, Jones BR, Esslemont DHB, Wiseman MS. A cross-sectional study of risk factors for obesity in cats in New Zealand. *Preventive Veterinary Medicine* 2000;46(3):183–196.
25. Zinn A. Unconvential wisdom about the obesity epidemic. *The American Journal of the Medical Sciences* 2010;340(6):481–491.
26. Farr OM, Li CS, Mantzoros CS. Central nervous system regulation of eating: Insights from human brain imaging. *Metabolism: Clinical and Experimental* 2016;65(5):699–713.
27. Allison MB, Myers MG. 20 years of leptin: Connecting leptin signaling to biological function. *Journal of Endocrinology* 2014;223(1):T25–T35.
28. Chan JL, Heist K, DePaoli AM, Veldhuis JD, Mantzoros CS. The role of falling leptin levels in the neuroendocrine and metabolic adaptation to short-term starvation in healthy men. *The Journal of Clinical Investigation* 2003;111(9):1409–1421.
29. Zhou Y, Rui L. Leptin signaling and leptin resistance. *Frontiers of Medicine* 2013;7(2):207–222.
30. Witzel A, Kirk C, Kania S et al. Relationship of adiponectin and its multimers to metabolic indices in cats during weight change. *Domestic Animal Endocrinology* 2015;53:70–77.
31. Backus R, Havel P, Gingerich R, Rogers Q. Relationship between serum leptin immunoreactivity and body fat mass as estimated by use of a novel gas-phase Fourier transform infrared spectroscopy deuterium dilution method in cats. *American Journal of Veterinary Research* 2000;61(7):796–801.
32. Appleton D, Rand J, Sunvold G. Plasma leptin concentrations in cats: Reference range, effect of weight gain and relationship with adiposity as measured by dual energy x-ray absorptiometry. *Journal of Feline Medicine & Surgery* 2000;2(4):191–199.

33. Martin LJM, Siliart B, Dumon HJW, Nguyen P. Spontaneous hormonal variations in male cats following gonadectomy. *Journal of Feline Medicine & Surgery* 2006;8(5):309–314.

34. Hoenig M, Thomaseth K, Waldron M, Ferguson DC. Insulin sensitivity, fat distribution, and adipocytokine response to different diets in lean and obese cats before and after weight loss. *American Journal of Physiology: Regulatory, Integrative and Comparative Physiology* 2007;292(1):R227–R234.

35. Park HJ, Lee S, Oh JH, Seo KW, Song KH. Leptin, adiponectin and serotonin levels in lean and obese dogs. *BMC Veterinary Research* 2014;10:113–114.

36. Wakshlag JJ, Struble AM, Levine CB, Bushey JJ, Laflamme DP, Long GM. The effects of weight loss on adipokines and markers of inflammation in dogs. *British Journal of Nutrition* 2011;106(Suppl 1):S11–S14.

37. Ueno H, Nakazato M. Mechanistic relationship between the vagal afferent pathway, central nervous system and peripheral organs in appetite regulation. *Journal of Diabetes Investigation* 2016;7(6):812–818.

38. Macht M. Characteristics of eating in anger, fear, sadness and joy. *Appetite* 1999;33(1):129–139.

39. Butte N, Cabellero B. Energy needs: Assessment and requirements. In: Shils M, editor, *Modern Nutrition in Health and Disease*. 10th ed. New York: Lippincott Williams & Wilkins; 2006, p. 136–147.

40. Ganong W. *Review of Medical Physiology*. 22nd ed. New York: Lange Medical Books/McGraw-Hill; 2005.

41. Kleiber, M. *The Fire of Life*. John Wiley & Sons, New York; 1961.

42. Hill RC. Challenges in measuring energy expenditure in companion animals: A clinician's perspective. *The Journal of Nutrition* 2006;136(7 Suppl):1967S–1972S.

43. López M, Alvarez CV, Nogueiras R, Diéguez C. Energy balance regulation by thyroid hormones at central level. *Trends in Molecular Medicine* 2013;19(7):418–427.

44. National Research Council (NRC). Energy. In: *Nutrient Requirements of Dogs and Cats*. Washington, D.C.: The National Academies Press; 2006, chap. 3.

45. Fain JN, Tagele BM, Cheema P, Madan AK, Tichansky DS. Release of 12 adipokines by adipose tissue, nonfat cells, and fat cells from obese women. *Obesity* 2010;18(5):890–896.

46. Ren J. Leptin and hyperleptinemia – From friend to foe for cardiovascular function. *Journal of Endocrinology* 2004;181(1):1–10.

47. Munzberg H, Myers Jr. MG. Molecular and anatomical determinants of central leptin resistance. *Nature Neuroscience* 2005;8(5):566–570.

48. Park S, Hong SM, Sung SR, Jung HK. Long-term effects of central leptin and resistin on body weight, insulin resistance, and beta-cell function and mass by the modulation of hypothalamic leptin and insulin signaling. *Endocrinology* 2007. doi:10.1210/en.2007-0754.

49. Sell H, Dietze-Schroeder D, Eckel J. The adipocyte-myocyte axis in insulin resistance. *Trends in Endocrinology & Metabolism* 2006;17(10):416–422.

50. Halaas JL, Gajiwala KS, Maffei M et al. Weight-reducing effects of the plasma protein encoded by the obese gene. *Science* 1995;269(5223):543–546.

51. Deng T, Lyon CJ, Bergin S, Caligiuri MA, Hsueh WA. Obesity, inflammation, and cancer. *Annual Review of Pathology* 2016;11:421–449.

52. Whitehead JP, Richards AA, Hickman IJ, Macdonald GA, Prins JB. Adiponectin: A key adipokine in the metabolic syndrome. *Diabetes, Obesity and Metabolism* 2006;8(3):264–280.

53. Arita Y, Kihara S, Ouchi N et al. Paradoxical decrease of an adipose-specific protein, adiponectin, in obesity. *Biochemical and Biophysical Research Communications* 1999;257(1):79–83.

54. Weyer C, Funahashi T, Tanaka S et al. Hypoadiponectinemia in obesity and type 2 diabetes: Close association with insulin resistance and hyperinsulinemia. *The Journal of Clinical Endocrinology and Metabolism* 2001;86(5):1930–1935.

55. Kantartzis K, Fritsche A, Tschritter O et al. The association between plasma adiponectin and insulin sensitivity in humans depends on obesity. *Obesity Research* 2005;13(10):1683–1691.

56. Tschritter O, Fritsche A, Thamer C et al. Plasma adiponectin concentrations predict insulin sensitivity of both glucose and lipid metabolism. *Diabetes* 2003;52(2):239–243.

57. Lindsay RS, Funahashi T, Hanson RL et al. Adiponectin and development of type 2 diabetes in the Pima Indian population. *Lancet* 2002;360(9326):57–58.

58. Yamamoto Y, Hirose H, Saito I, Nishikai K, Saruta T. Adiponectin, an adipocyte-derived protein, predicts future insulin resistance: Two-year follow-up study in Japanese population. *The Journal of Clinical Endocrinology and Metabolism* 2004;89(1):87–90.

59. Snehalatha C, Mukesh B, Simon M, Viswanathan V, Haffner SM, Ramachandran A. Plasma adiponectin is an independent predictor of type 2 diabetes in Asian Indians. *Diabetes Care* 2003;26(12):3226–3229.

60. Spranger J, Kroke A, Mohlig M et al. Adiponectin and protection against type 2 diabetes mellitus. *Lancet* 2003;361(9353):226–228.

61. Greenberg AS, Obin MS. Obesity and the role of adipose tissue in inflammation and metabolism. *The American Journal of Clinical Nutrition* 2006;83(2):461S–465S.

62. Ouchi N, Walsh K. Adiponectin as an anti-inflammatory factor. *Clinica Chimica Acta* 2007;380(12):24–30.

63. Hoenig M, Jordan ET, Glushka J et al. Effect of macronutrients, age, and obesity on 6- and 24-h postprandial glucose metabolism in cats. *American Journal of Physiology: Regulatory, Integrative and Comparative Physiology* 2011;301(6):R1798–R1807.

64. Ellekilde M, Selfjord E, Larsen CS et al. Transfer of gut microbiota from lean and obese mice to antibiotic-treated mice. *Scientific Reports* 2014;4:5922. doi:10.1038/srep05922.

65. Ishioka K, Omachi A, Sasaki N, Kimura K, Saito M. Feline adiponectin: Molecular structures and plasma concentrations in obese cats. *The Journal of Veterinary Medical Science* 2009;71(2):189–5194.
66. Muranaka S, Mori N, Hatano Y et al. Obesity induced changes to plasma adiponectin concentration and cholesterol lipoprotein composition profile in cats. *Research in Veterinary Science* 2011;91(3):358–361.
67. Tvarijonaviciute A, Ceron JJ, Holden SL, Morris PJ, Biourge V, German AJ. Effects of weight loss in obese cats on biochemical analytes related to inflammation and glucose homeostasis. *Domestic Animal Endocrinology* 2012;42(3):129–141.
68. Bjornvad CR, Rand JS, Tan HY et al. Obesity and sex influence insulin resistance and total and multimer adiponectin levels in adult neutered domestic shorthair client-owned cats. *Domestic Animal Endocrinology* 2014;47:55–64. doi:10.1016/j.domaniend.2013.11.006.
69. Coradini M, Rand JS, Morton JM, Arai T, Ishioka K, Rawlings JM. Fat mass, and not diet, has a large effect on postprandial leptin but not on adiponectin concentrations in cats. *Domestic Animal Endocrinology* 2013;45(2):79–88.
70. Prince AL, Chu DM, Seferovic MD, Antony KM, Ma J, Aagaard KM. The perinatal microbiome and pregnancy: Moving beyond the vaginal microbiome. *Cold Spring Harbor Perspectives in Medicine* 2015;5(6). doi:10.1101/cshperspect.a023051.
71. Brunson BL, Zhong Q, Clarke KJ et al. Serum concentrations of adiponectin and characterization of adiponectin protein complexes in dogs. *American Journal of Veterinary Research* 2007;68(1):57–62.
72. Ishioka K, Omachi A, Sagawa M et al. Canine adiponectin: cDNA structure, mRNA expression in adipose tissues and reduced plasma levels in obesity. *Research in Veterinary Science* 2006;80(2):127–132.
73. Bäckhed F, Manchester JK, Semenkovich CF, Gordon JI. Mechanisms underlying the resistance to diet-induced obesity in germ-free mice. *Proceedings of the National Academy of Sciences USA* 2007;104(3):979–984. doi:10.1073/pnas.0605374104.
74. Tvarijonaviciute A, Martínez-Subiela S, Ceron JJ. Validation of 2 commercially available enzyme-linked immunosorbent assays for adiponectin determination in canine serum samples. *Canadian Journal of Veterinary Research* 2010;74(4):279–285.
75. German AJ, Hervera M, Hunter L et al. Improvement in insulin resistance and reduction in plasma inflammatory adipokines after weight loss in obese dogs. *Domestic Animal Endocrinology* 2009;37(4):214–226.
76. Verkest KR, Fleeman LM, Rand JS, Morton JM. Evaluation of beta-cell sensitivity to glucose and first-phase insulin secretion in obese dogs. *American Journal of Veterinary Research* 2011;72(3):357–366.
77. Verkest KR, Rose FJ, Fleeman LM et al. Adiposity and adiponectin in dogs: Investigation of causes of discrepant results between two studies. *Domestic Animal Endocrinology* 2011;41(1):35–41.
78. Alang N, Colleen RK. Weight gain after fecal microbiota transplantation. *Open Forum Infectious Diseases* 2015;2(1). doi:10.1093/ofid/ofv004.

79. Weisberg SP, McCann D, Desai M, Rosenbaum M, Leibel RL, Ferrante AW. Obesity is associated with macrophage accumulation in adipose tissue. *Journal of Clinical Investigation* 2003;112:1796–1808.

80. Cawthorn WP, Sethi JK. TNF-[alpha] and adipocyte biology. *FEBS Letters* 2008;582(1):117–131.

81. Fain JN, Bahouth SW, Madan AK. TNF[alpha] release by the nonfat cells of human adipose tissue. *International Journal of Obesity and Related Metabolic Disorders* 2004;28(4):616–622.

82. Ryden M, Arner P. Tumour necrosis factor-alpha in human adipose tissue – From signalling mechanisms to clinical implications. *Journal of Internal Medicine* 2007;262(4):431–438.

83. Mohamed-Ali V, Goodrick S, Rawesh A et al. Subcutaneous adipose tissue releases interleukin-6, but not tumor necrosis factor-alpha, *in vivo*. *The Journal of Clinical Endocrinology and Metabolism* 1997;82(12):4196–4200.

84. Hotamisligil GS, Shargill NS, Spiegelman BM. Adipose expression of tumor necrosis factor-alpha: Direct role in obesity-linked insulin resistance. *Science* 1993;259(5091):87–91.

85. Mandalia A, Ward A, Tauxe W, Kraft CS, Dhere T. Fecal transplant is as effective and safe in immunocompromised as non-immunocompromised patients for *Clostridium difficile*. *International Journal of Colorectal Disease* 2015;September. doi:10.1007/s00384-015-2396-2.

86. Hoenig M, McGoldrick JB, deBeer M, Demacker PNM, Ferguson DC. Activity and tissue-specific expression of lipases and tumor-necrosis factor alpha in lean and obese cats. *Domestic Animal Endocrinology* 2006;30(4):333–344.

87. Stephens JM, Lee J, Pilch PF. Tumor necrosis factor-alpha-insulin resistance in 3T3–L1 adipocytes is accompanied by a loss of insulin receptor substrate-1 and GLUT4 expression without a loss of insulin receptor-mediated signal transduction. *Journal of Biological Chemistry* 1997;272(2):971–976.

88. Qi C, Pekala PH. Tumor necrosis factor-alpha induced insulin resistance in adipocytes. *Proceedings of the Society for Experimental Biology and Medicine* 2000;223(2):128–135.

89. Peraldi P, Xu M, Spiegelman BM. Thiazolidinediones block tumor necrosis factor-alpha induced inhibition of insulin signaling. *Journal of Clinical Investigation* 1997;100(7):1863–1869.

90. Memon RA, Feingold KR, Moser AH, Fuller J, Grunfeld C. Regulation of fatty acid transport protein and fatty acid translocase mRNA levels by endotoxin and cytokines. *American Journal of Physiology* 1998;274:E210–E217.

91. Kita A, Yamasaki H, Kuwahara H et al. Identification of the promoter region required for human adiponectin gene transcription: Association with CCAAT/enhancer binding protein-[beta] and tumor necrosis factor-[alpha]. *Biochemical and Biophysical Research Communications* 2005;331(2):484–490.

92. Kim KY, Kim JK, Jeon JH, Yoon SR, Choi I, Yang Y. c-Jun N-terminal kinase is involved in the suppression of adiponectin expression by TNF-[alpha] in 3T3–L1 adipocytes. *Biochemical and Biophysical Research Communications* 2005;327(2):460–467.

93. Wolin KY, Carson K, Colditz GA. Obesity and cancer. *The Oncologist* 2010;15(6):556–565.

94. Vainio H, Kaaks R, Bianchini F. Weight control and physical activity in cancer prevention: International evaluation of the evidence. *European Journal of Cancer Prevention* 2002;(11 Suppl 2):S94–S100.

95. Janesick A, Blumberg B. Endocrine disrupting chemicals and the developmental programming of adipogenesis and obesity. *Birth Defects Research (Part C)* 2011;93:34–50.

96. Spalding KL, Arner E, Westermark PO et al. Dynamics of fat cell turnover in humans. *Nature* 2008;453:783–787.

97. Ye J, Gimble J. Regulation of stem cell differentiation in adipose tissue by chronic inflammation. *Clinical and Experimental Pharmacology and Physiology* 2011;38:872–878.

98. Assim A, Sallam A, Sallam R. Reactive oxygen species in health and disease. *Journal of Biomedicine and Biotechnology* 2012;2012:1–2.

99. Dikalov SI, Nazarewicz RR. Angiotensin II-induced production of mitochondrial reactive oxygen species: Potential mechanisms and relevance for cardiovascular disease. *Antioxidants & Redox Signaling* 2013;19(10):1085–1094.

100. Bäckhed F, Ding H, Wang T et al. The gut microbiota as an environmental factor that regulates fat storage. *Proceedings of the National Academy of Sciences* 2004;101(44):15718–15723.

101. Ley RE, Turnbaugh PJ, Klein S, Gordon JI. Microbial ecology: Human gut microbes associated with obesity. *Nature* 2006;444(7122):1022–1023. doi:10.1038/4441022a.

102. Turnbaugh PJ, Ley RE, Hamady M, Fraser-Liggett CM, Knight R, Gordon JI. The human microbiome project. *Nature* 2007;449(7164):804–810.

103. Ley RE, Peterson DA, Gordon JI. Ecological and evolutionary forces shaping microbial diversity in the human intestine. *Cell* 2006;124(4):837–848. doi:10.1016/j.cell.2006.02.017.

104. Bäckhed F, Ley RE, Sonnenburg JL, Peterson DA, Gordon JI. Host-bacterial mutualism in the human intestine. *Science* 2005; 307(5717):1915–1920.

105. Turnbaugh PJ, Ley RE, Mahowald MA, Magrini V, Mardis ER, Gordon JI. An obesity-associated gut microbiome with increased capacity for energy harvest. *Nature* 2006;444(7122):1027–1031.

106. Turnbaugh PJ, Hamady M, Yatsunenko T et al. A core gut microbiome in obese and lean twins. *Nature* 2009;457(7228):480–484.

107. Handl S, German AJ, Holden SL et al. Faecal microbiota in lean and obese dogs. *FEMS Microbiology Ecology* 2013;84(2):332–343. doi:10.1111/1574-6941.12067.

108. Park H-J, Lee S-E, Kim H-B, Isaacson RE, Seo K-W, Song K-H. Association of obesity with serum leptin, adiponectin, and serotonin and gut microflora in Beagle dogs. *Journal of Veterinary Internal Medicine/ American College of Veterinary Internal Medicine* 2015;29(1):43–50. doi:10.1111/jvim.12455.

109. De Filippo C, Cavalieri D, Di Paola M et al. Impact of diet in shaping gut microbiota revealed by a comparative study in children from Europe and Rural Africa. *Proceedings of the National Academy of Sciences* 2010;107(33):14691–14696.

110. Sankar SA, Lagier J-C, Pontarotti P, Raoult D, Fournier P-E. The human gut microbiome, a taxonomic conundrum. *Systematic and Applied Microbiology* 2015;38(4):276–286. doi:10.1016/j.syapm.2015.03.004.

111. Samuel BS, Gordon JI. A humanized gnotobiotic mouse model of host-archaeal-bacterial mutualism. *Proceedings of the National Academy of Sciences* 2006;103(26):10011–10016. doi:10.1073/pnas.0602187103.

112. McNeil NI. The contribution of the large intestine to energy supplies in man. *American Journal of Clinical Nutrition* 1984;39(2):338–342.

113. Li M, Gu D, Xu N et al. Gut carbohydrate metabolism instead of fat metabolism regulated by gut microbes mediates high-fat diet-induced obesity. *Beneficial Microbes* 2014;5(3):335–344. doi:10.3920/BM2013.0071.

114. Samuel BS, Shaito A, Motoike T et al. Effects of the gut microbiota on host adiposity are modulated by the short-chain fatty-acid binding G protein-coupled receptor, Gpr41. *Proceedings of the National Academy of Sciences* 2008;105(43):16767–16772. doi:10.1073/pnas.0808567105.

115. Middelbos IS, Boler BMV, Qu A, White BA, Swanson KS, Fahey GC. Phylogenetic characterization of fecal microbial communities of dogs fed diets with or without supplemental dietary fiber using 454 pyrosequencing. *PLOS ONE* 2010;5(3):e9768–e9769. doi:10.1371/journal.pone.0009768.

116. Qiao Y, Sun J, Xia S, Tang X, Shi Y, Le G. Effects of resveratrol on gut microbiota and fat storage in a mouse model with high-fat-induced obesity. *Food & Function* 2014;5(6):1241–1249. doi:10.1039/c3fo60630a.

117. Marques TM, Wall R, O'Sullivan O et al. Dietary trans-10, Cis-12–conjugated linoleic acid alters fatty acid metabolism and microbiota composition in mice. *The British Journal of Nutrition* 2015;113(5):728–738. doi:10.1017/S0007114514004206.

118. Cluny NL, Eller LK, Keenan CM, Reimer RA, Sharkey KA. Interactive effects of oligofructose and obesity predisposition on gut hormones and microbiota in diet-induced obese rats. *Obesity (Silver Spring, MD)* 2015;23(4):769–778. doi:10.1002/oby.21017.

119. Duca FA, Sakar Y, Lepage P et al. Replication of obesity and associated signaling pathways through transfer of microbiota from obese-prone rats. *Diabetes* 2014;63(5):1624–1636. doi:10.2337/db13–1526.

120. Jewell DE, Toll PW, Azain MJ, Lewis RD, Edwards GL. Fiber but not conjugated linoleic acid influences adiposity in dogs. *Veterinary Therapeutics* 2006;7(2):78–85.
121. Grześkowiak Ł, Endo A, Beasley S, Salminen S. Microbiota and probiotics in canine and feline welfare. *Anaerobe* 2015;34(August):14–23. doi:10.1016/j.anaerobe.2015.04.002.
122. Silva BC, Jung LRC, Sandes SHC et al. In vitro assessment of functional properties of lactic acid bacteria isolated from faecal microbiota of healthy dogs for potential use as probiotics. *Beneficial Microbes* 2013;4(3):267–275. doi:10.3920/BM2012.0048.
123. Garcia-Mazcorro JF, Lanerie DJ, Dowd SE et al. Effect of a multi-species synbiotic formulation on fecal bacterial microbiota of healthy cats and dogs as evaluated by pyrosequencing. *FEMS Microbiology Ecology* 2011;78(3):542–554. doi:10.1111/j.1574–6941.2011.01185.x.
124. Luoto R, Kalliomäki M, Laitinen K, Isolauri E. The impact of perinatal probiotic intervention on the development of overweight and obesity: Follow-up study from birth to 10 years. *International Journal of Obesity* 2010;34(10):1531–1537. doi:10.1038/ijo.2010.50.
125. Luoto R, Laitinen K, Nermes M, Isolauri E. Impact of maternal probiotic-supplemented dietary counselling on pregnancy outcome and prenatal and postnatal growth: A double-blind, placebo-controlled study. *The British Journal of Nutrition* 2010;103(12):1792–1799. doi:10.1017/S0007114509993898.
126. Cengiz Ö, Köksal BH, Tatlı O et al. Effect of dietary probiotic and high stocking density on the performance, carcass yield, gut microflora, and stress indicators of broilers. *Poultry Science* 2015;94(10):2395–2403. doi:10.3382/ps/pev194.
127. Zbinden A, Zbinden R, Berger C, Arlettaz R. Case series of *Bifidobacterium longum* bacteremia in three preterm infants on probiotic therapy. *Neonatology* 2015;107(1):56–59. doi:10.1159/000367985.
128. Eren Z, Gurol Y, Sonmezoglu M, Eren HS, Celik G, Kantarci G. Saccharomyces cerevisiae fungemia in an elderly patient following probiotic treatment. *Mikrobiyoloji Bülteni* 2014;48(2):351–355.
129. Suchodolski JS, Dowd SE, Westermarck E et al. The effect of the macrolide antibiotic tylosin on microbial diversity in the canine small intestine as demonstrated by massive parallel 16S rRNA gene sequencing. *BMC Microbiology* 2009;9:210. doi:10.1186/1471-2180-9-210.
130. Procter TD, Pearl DL, Finley RL et al. A cross-sectional study examining the prevalence and risk factors for anti-microbial-resistant generic escherichia coli in domestic dogs that frequent dog parks in three cities in South-Western Ontario, Canada. *Zoonoses and Public Health* 2014;61(4):250–259. doi:10.1111/zph.12064.
131. Peter D, Sørensen AH, Guardabassi L. Monitoring of antimicrobial resistance in healthy dogs: First report of canine ampicillin-resistant enterococcus faecium clonal complex 17. *Veterinary Microbiology* 2008;132(1-2):190–196. doi:10.1016/j.vetmic.2008.04.026.

132. Eiseman B, Silen W, Bascom GS, Kauvar AJ. Fecal enema as an adjunct in the treatment of pseudomembranous enterocolitis. *Surgery* 1958;44(5):854–859.

133. Brandt LJ. Fecal microbiota transplant: Respice, adspice, prospice. *Journal of Clinical Gastroenterology* 2015;49(Suppl 1 December):S65–S68. doi:10.1097/MCG.0000000000000346.

134. Borody T, Fischer M, Mitchell S, Campbell J. Fecal microbiota transplantation in gastrointestinal disease: 2015 update and the road ahead. *Expert Review of Gastroenterology & Hepatology*. 2015;September:1–13. doi:10.1586/17474124.2015.1086267.

Pathophysiology of obesity: Comorbidities and anesthetic considerations

VALERIE J. PARKER, ELIZABETH ORCUTT, AND LYDIA LOVE

3.1 INTRODUCTION

The associations between body weight and many comorbidities have been studied. This chapter will review some of these relationships in dogs and cats as well as provide recommendations for management. In addition, perianesthetic management of obese patients will be considered.

3.2 OBESITY AND LIFE SPAN

The effect of body weight on life span has been evaluated in dogs. In a lifetime study of 24 pairs of Labrador retriever littermates from 7 litters, dogs in the restricted calorie group were fed 25% less than the control calorie group (1). Dogs in the restricted group maintained a body condition score (BCS) of 4–5/9, compared to dogs in the control group that maintained a BCS of 6–7/9. This long-term caloric restriction and maintenance of lean BCS resulted in a 1.8-year longer median life span in the restricted group ($P < 0.01$) (1). Metabolic phenotypes of these two groups were determined by use of orthogonal projections to latent structures discriminant analysis (OPLS-DA). There were a few significant differences between groups (e.g., differences in energy and lipoprotein metabolism), supporting the notion that caloric restriction is associated with decreased risk factors for several comorbidities (e.g., obesity, diabetes mellitus) commonly seen with advancing age (2).

The effects of height and weight on life span were evaluated in 718 dogs representing 77 American Kennel Club (AKC) breeds (3). There were significant inverse relationships between life span and weight and height ($r = -0.68$ and $r = -0.60$, respectively; $P < 0.05$). In regression analysis, 58.5% variability in life span could be accounted for by differences in height and weight in otherwise healthy dogs. Ultimately, the authors concluded that smaller dogs that weighed less typically lived longer than the larger, heavier counterparts. One primary limitation to this study was that it did not evaluate BCS. There are no published studies to date evaluating the relationship between body weight and life span in cats. Overall, these studies in dogs suggest that a regular part of preventative care for veterinary patients should include prevention of overweight and obesity.

3.3 OBESITY PARADOX

Despite obesity predisposing people and animals to certain conditions, the "obesity paradox" relates to improved survival once chronic illnesses are diagnosed. This paradox is well established in people with various conditions (4–7). Most studies of the obesity paradox in people have shown a linear relationship between body weight and survival (8,9), although some have demonstrated a U- or J-shaped curve, with people having the highest body weight also having decreased survival (10,11).

In veterinary medicine, the obesity paradox has been investigated in dogs and cats with cancer (12), heart failure (13,14), and chronic kidney disease (CKD) (15,16). Dogs with heart failure that gained body weight had longer survival times compared to those that lost or maintained body weight (13). In CKD dogs, those with a thin BCS (≤3/9) had significantly shorter survival than dogs with a BCS ≥4 (15). Additionally, cats with a body weight of <4.2 kg at the time of CKD diagnosis had a significantly shorter survival time compared to cats ≥4.2 kg (16).

In cats with cancer, both body weight and BCS were significantly associated with survival (12). In cats with heart failure, cats with low body weight had shorter survival times compared to cats with moderate body weights. However, cats with the highest body weights also had reduced survival times, suggesting a U-shaped relationship between body weight and survival (4). Similar findings were found in cats with CKD; a J-shaped survival curve was documented (Figure 3.1) (16).

The mechanism by which overweight and obesity exert a protective effect in these varied diseases is not completely understood, but several theories are

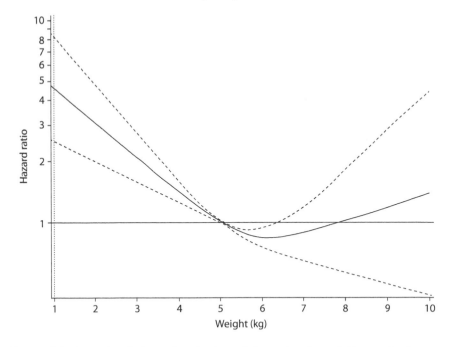

Figure 3.1 Hazard ratio based on body weight at the time of diagnosis of chronic kidney disease of 569 cats. Dotted lines indicate the 95% confidence interval. Cats with the lowest and highest body weights at the time of diagnosis of CKD have shorter survival times than cats with more moderate body weights ($P < 0.0001$). (Adapted from Freeman LM et al., *Journal of Veterinary Internal Medicine* 2016;30:1661–1666.)

described. It is likely multifactorial, related to altered adipokine (adipose tissue hormones) profiles, neurohormonal alterations and medications used to treat concurrent diseases. One important explanation for the obesity paradox is that obesity reflects higher muscle mass, or lack of cachexia, since people with obesity not only have more adipose tissue compared to lean people but also have more lean body mass (7). The detrimental effects of muscle loss in a variety of diseases are well documented (17). Therefore, this extra lean body mass associated with obesity may provide greater reserve in CKD or other catabolic diseases.

Ultimately this paradox should be considered in overweight animals with comorbid conditions when determining if weight loss should be a goal, and if so, how much weight loss should be attained. For example, a dog with a BCS of 6/9 and a diagnosis of congestive heart failure secondary to chronic valvular disease may be fed to maintain its current body weight rather than fed to achieve a BCS of 4–5/9.

3.4 ENDOCRINE DISEASE

3.4.1 Diabetes mellitus

Diabetes mellitus (DM) is a common endocrinopathy affecting dogs and cats. In dogs, diabetes more closely resembles human type 1 DM, in which β-cell destruction causes an absolute insulin deficiency. The majority of feline DM resembles human type 2 DM in which insulin resistance occurs in the liver, muscle, and adipose tissues, progressing to β-cell failure and insulin dependency.

3.4.2 Canine diabetes mellitus

Being overweight was positively associated with a diagnosis of DM in dogs presenting to first-opinion practices in the United Kingdom (18). However, causal evidence of a direct link from obesity to the development of DM in the dog has not been established. Proopiomelanocortin (POMC) gene deletion in Labrador retrievers is associated with increased appetite and risk of obesity (19). Researchers investigating a potential link between POMC gene deletion and the development of DM were unable to find an association in dogs (20).

Obesity presents a challenge in the management of diabetic dogs. Obesity in the dog has been shown to result in insulin resistance (21). Although this has not been shown to result in type 2 DM, this will impact glycemic control. Insulin sensitivity in lean dogs was 58% greater than overweight dogs (2). Additionally, dogs with a body weight gain of approximately 43% had significantly higher basal insulinemia and insulin resistance (22). Further affecting both insulin resistance and glycemic control, obesity induces a state of chronic low-grade inflammation. Weight loss in overweight dogs decreases insulin resistance and inflammatory markers, specifically tumor necrosis factor-α (TNF-α), haptoglobin, and C-reactive protein concentrations (23). A marker of glycemic control in dogs is maintenance of body weight. While it is important to evaluate diabetic regulation accurately, patients presenting in a state of obesity should have a dietary plan to help with controlled weight management in conjunction with appropriate medical management.

3.4.3 Feline diabetes mellitus

Obesity is the most important risk factor for the development of DM in the cat. Cats with an obese body condition are 3.9 times as likely to have DM than cats with an ideal BCS leading to decreased insulin sensitivity (24). Insulin resistance can occur at just 10% over a cat's lean body weight (25). A 30% reduction in insulin sensitivity is associated with a kilogram increase in body weight (26). The development of DM in overweight domestic shorthair cats has been linked to a polymorphism of the melanocortin 4 receptor (MC4R) gene, which has roles in energy balance and appetite (27). Adipose tissue can produce adipokine hormones that can influence energy balance and glucose metabolism. The adipokine adiponectin is negatively correlated to fat mass and increases insulin sensitivity (26,28). In another study, adiponectin concentrations did not differ significantly between lean, overweight, and obese cats (29). Zapata et al. found lower adiponectin in diabetic cats when compared to lean and overweight cats (30). Further, this study found increased concentrations of leptin, an adipokine positively correlated to fat mass, in diabetic and overweight cats when compared to lean cats.

Intake of dry extruded food has been associated with obesity and/or the development of DM in the cat (31,32). Dry extruded food typically has a higher carbohydrate content than the natural diet of cats (33). Due to the nature of these studies, a causal relationship between dietary carbohydrate intake and the development of obesity and diabetes mellitus is not established. Limitations such as recall bias, owner reporting of BCS, and lack of macronutrient and dietary intake may have confounded the result of these studies. The role of dietary carbohydrates in feline obesity and DM is beyond the scope of this book chapter, but the reader is directed to a review article by Verbrugghe and Hesta for further discussion (34). Excess caloric intake and ad libitum feeding of dry food are more likely contributors to the development of obesity and diabetes mellitus in the cat.

Although the role of dietary carbohydrates in the development of DM is unclear, there is evidence to support low-carbohydrate diets for the treatment of DM (35–37). Cats fed a low-carbohydrate, low-fiber diet were more likely to have better glycemic control and achieve diabetic remission than cats fed a moderate-carbohydrate, high-fiber diet (35). The two study diets contained different ingredients and macronutrient content, including protein and fat, which may have influenced the results. The use of a low-carbohydrate, high-protein diet reduced the insulin requirement in cats when switched from a high-fiber diet (37). Diet recommendations should also include a recommendation for weight loss in obese diabetic patients to improve peripheral insulin sensitivity and promote diabetic remission. Weight loss has been shown to normalize insulin sensitivity in cats (26).

3.4.4 Hyperadrenocorticism

Hyperadrenocorticism (HAC) is a common endocrinopathy affecting middle aged to older dogs. The development of visceral obesity and abdominal distension is a classic clinical sign of HAC. Visceral adiposity and HAC may be associated with changes in adipokine and hormone production. Overweight dogs with pituitary-dependent hyperadrenocorticism (PDH) had higher concentrations of leptin and insulin compared to overweight dogs without PDH (38). Leptin concentrations were linearly associated with serum cortisol concentrations in this same study. It has been suggested in people (39) that hyperleptinemia has inflammatory, thrombotic, and oxidative effects that may play a role in the progression and occurrence of complications related to HAC; however, further studies are needed to evaluate this relationship in the dog. Following treatment with trilostane, concentrations of insulin and leptin were reduced but still higher when compared to controls, which may be the result of intermittent periods of hypercortisolism and higher visceral fat content when compared to controls (38). Changes in adiponectin are inconsistent between studies with one study reporting decreased concentrations in dogs with PDH and another reporting no difference when compared to controls with a similar BCS (38,40). The latter study reported this lack of significance may be due to the small study population.

Treatment of HAC with trilostane resulted in significant decreases in body weight and BCS in overweight dogs (38). Changes to diet or purposeful weight management were not reported in this study. Weight reduction in addition to medical management of HAC to reduce visceral adiposity and potentially improve control of disease has not been investigated. Hyperlipidemia is often associated with HAC in addition to visceral adiposity, therefore diet change to aid in the management of this disease is reasonable.

3.4.5 Hypothyroidism

Thyroid hormone is necessary for all normal metabolic functions throughout the body, therefore hypothyroidism affects the metabolic function of almost all organ systems. Clinical signs seen with metabolic derangements associated with hypothyroidism include lethargy, exercise intolerance, and weight gain without increased appetite or food intake. Energy expenditure in hypothyroid dogs was noted to be 15% less compared with normal dogs that returned to normal after treatment (41). Achieving weight loss in hypothyroid dogs first should focus on restoration of euthyroidism to improve energy expenditure. If desired weight loss is not achieved with normalization of thyroid hormone alone, further nutritional management is recommended.

3.4.6 Hyperlipidemia

Hyperlipidemia in the dog and cat refers to the increase of plasma or serum cholesterol and/or triglycerides. Causes of fasting hyperlipidemia can either be a primary disorder of lipid metabolism or secondary to other disease processes with secondary hyperlipidemias being more common. Obesity is an important secondary cause of hyperlipidemia. Concentrations of cholesterol and/or triglycerides are increased in obese dogs when compared to lean controls (22,42,43). Plasma cholesterol and triglyceride concentrations were significantly higher in obese versus lean cats (44). In a more recent study, nondiabetic, client-owned overweight and obese cats had higher serum triglycerides but not cholesterol when compared to lean cats (45). In obese beagle dogs, switching from an adult maintenance diet to a low energy-density diet with a reduced caloric intake results in improved plasma cholesterol and triglyceride concentrations even before significant weight loss occurred (43). Diet change with subsequent weight loss is also reported to improve cholesterol and triglyceride concentrations in the dog (46,47).

Recognition of fasting hyperlipidemia in dogs is important due to its association with clinically relevant diseases such as pancreatitis, hepatobiliary disease, ocular disease, insulin resistance, and atherosclerosis (48). Dyslipidemia in obese cats is also associated with insulin resistance and diabetes mellitus (44,45,49,50). Treatment of secondary causes of hyperlipidemia should focus on resolution or control of the underlying condition, therefore weight loss is recommended for patients with hyperlipidemia and obesity. Reduction of the patient's fat intake should also be considered, particularly in patients with severe, persistent, or primary hyperlipidemias. Studies evaluating the levels of dietary fat for reducing hyperlipidemias are lacking in the dog and cat. Decreasing a patient's fat intake may be relative to their current intake. In the dog, the authors recommend feeding a diet containing ≤ 25 grams of fat per 1000 kcals.

3.5 CARDIOVASCULAR AND RESPIRATORY DISEASE

Alterations in cardiovascular and respiratory physiology can occur in the obese state. The reader is referred to Section 3.9 for further discussion on pathophysiology.

3.5.1 Congestive heart failure and cardiovascular disease

Congestive heart failure (CHF) is typically associated with a catabolic state that results in the loss of lean body mass contributing to cardiac cachexia. Many patients presenting with CHF are overweight or obese. Forty-one percent of dogs and 37% of cats presenting with CHF were either overweight or obese (13,14). In canine CHF, elevated levels of leptin have been detected (51). There was no correlation between leptin concentration and BCS although no obese dogs (BCS $\geq 8/9$) were included in this study. Elevated leptin concentrations may contribute to the development of cardiac cachexia due to increases in metabolic rate and association with pro-inflammatory cytokines and catecholamines. Survival times may be improved in patients above an ideal body condition termed the "obesity paradox" (see Section 3.3). A study of survival in dogs with CHF failed to demonstrate a significant association with BCS; however, weight change was significantly associated with survival with dogs gaining weight surviving the longest (13). A similar study in cats with CHF found a U-shaped relationship between body weight and survival with reduced survival times in cats with the lowest and highest body weight (14).

Obesity is not associated with the development of coronary artery disease in the dog or cat as it is in people (52). Dogs and cats lack significant activity of the enzyme cholesterol ester transfer protein (CETP) responsible for the transfer to cholesterol esters from high-density lipoproteins (HDL) to very low-density lipoproteins (VLDL), and low-density lipoproteins (LDL). This results in the transfer of cholesterol esters to the liver by HDL molecules rather than the peripheral tissues.

3.5.2 Hypertension

The association between canine obesity and hypertension is debatable. Although a few studies have documented that obesity may induce hypertension (53,54), this finding is not universal. In one study where there was no association between BCS and hypertension, the authors suggested that it is possible that obese dogs are more likely to have comorbidities that may induce hypertension (e.g., cardiac disease, endocrinopathies) (55). Most authors have concluded that the effect, if present is typically minor and does not usually require specific antihypertensive therapy (56,57). No association in cats has been documented between obesity and hypertension (49).

3.5.3 Collapsing trachea

Many patients presenting with collapsing trachea are overweight or obese. The median BCS in dogs diagnosed with collapsing trachea was 7/9 with 64% of dogs reported as overweight or obese (58). Another study investigating the outcome between two therapeutic procedures in 103 dogs reported a median BCS of 7/9 in each group (59). Obesity is a secondary factor in initiating clinical signs and contributing to the progression of tracheal collapse (60). Weight loss is considered an essential part of medical management to improve clinical signs, although no studies are currently available to evaluate this recommendation in the dog (60). Intrathoracic adipose tissue can reduce thoracic wall compliance and thoracic movement reducing respiratory function. Thoracic wall compliance can be improved by reducing excess adipose tissue including intra-abdominal and extrathoracic deposits. Weight loss depends primarily on dietary management for these patients, as many cannot exercise safely without exacerbating clinical signs.

3.6 RENAL AND URINARY DISEASE

3.6.1 Renal disease

Body condition score may be a risk factor for development, as well as progression, of kidney disease. In a retrospective study to identify risk factors associated with diagnosis of CKD, cats with a BCS of 1–2/5 were found to be at higher risk than those with an ideal or high BCS (61). Cats with a body weight >4.2 kg at diagnosis had a significantly longer survival time than cats with a body weight <4.2 kg at diagnosis (16).

In dogs, despite evidence that having a BCS ≥4/9 may offer some longevity benefit (15), obesity has been shown to induce adverse renal effects. Experimentally induced obesity in dogs increased arterial blood pressure and activation of the renin–angiotensin system. It caused glomerular hyperfiltration and histologic changes consistent with glomerular injury (62). It has yet to be determined if obesity is a significant risk factor in dogs and cats for development of naturally occurring renal disease.

One study evaluated the impact of weight loss in 37 obese dogs on indicators of renal function (63). After weight loss, urea and urine specific gravity were increased. Urine protein:creatinine (UPC) ratio, urine albumin:creatinine (UAC) ratio, and creatinine were decreased after weight loss. Three novel biomarkers of renal function (homocysteine, cystatin C, and clusterin) all decreased with weight loss. The authors concluded that canine obesity could result in subclinical alterations in renal function, which can improve with weight loss (63). In contrast, another study found no association between UPC and BCS in dogs (BCS 4–5/9 versus BCS >6/9) (64). This study was unable to differentiate between overweight and obese BCS due to the limited sample size. If an overweight/obese animal has significant proteinuria, it may be warranted to consider use of a lower protein low calorie diet to achieve weight loss while not exacerbating proteinuria.

3.6.2 Urinary disease

Increasing body weight has been documented as a risk factor for feline lower urinary tract disease (FLUTD), a syndrome that encompasses feline idiopathic cystitis (FIC), urolithiasis, urinary tract infections (UTI), urethral obstruction (UO), and neoplasia (65–67). This association has been reported most in cases of FIC (65,66), possibly related to findings from another study indicating that low activity level was associated with development of FLUTD (68). There was no association between body weight and risk of FLUTD in another epidemiologic study (69). Increased body weight was also shown to be a risk factor for UO as compared to control cats (70).

The relationship between BCS and calcium oxalate (CaOx) urolithiasis has been studied in dogs. One study found that dogs with CaOx uroliths had a significantly greater median BCS (6/9; range, 4–7/9) than case controls (5/9; range, 4–7/9); however, the proportion of overweight cases in both groups did not significantly differ and no obese dogs were included (BCS ≥8/9) (71). Despite a well-documented relationship between obesity and urinary incontinence in women (72), there are no published reports of this association in veterinary medicine. Increased prevalence of asymptomatic bacteriuria in morbidly obese dogs (body fat >45% as assessed by dual energy absorptiometry) has also been reported (73).

3.7 ORTHOPEDIC AND NEUROLOGIC DISEASE

3.7.1 Orthopedic disease

Obesity is postulated to be a risk factor for development of osteoarthritis (OA). It is possible that inflammatory mediators secreted by body fat may contribute to onset and progression of disease (74,75). In 92 Labrador retrievers of varying body compositions, fasting plasma interleukin-6 (IL-6) and monocyte chemotactic protein-1 (MCP-1) concentrations were associated with increasing BCS, highlighting the relationship between obesity and chronic inflammation (76). In diet-induced obese rats, OA was associated with greater body fat but not necessarily body mass (77).

Several canine studies have examined the relationship between body weight and degenerative joint disease (DJD) and OA. One of the earliest studies to document this relationship showed that obesity was associated with articular and/or locomotor problems. Although this study did not use objective measures to document OA, it did lay some groundwork for future studies (78). In a lifetime study of 48 Labrador retriever dogs, there was no difference in frequency of elbow OA in dogs fed 25% fewer calories than their control-fed pair mates (79). The severity of elbow OA was significantly worse in the control-fed dogs at 6 years of age, but not at 8 years and end of life. In the same dogs, caloric restriction was associated with delayed radiographic development of hip OA. The median age at which OA was detected was 12 years for the calorie-restricted dogs versus 6 years for their control-fed pair mates (80). In another study, body weight was a significant risk factor for radiographic evidence of DJD in 15,742 dogs representing 4 large dog breeds (golden retrievers, Labrador retrievers, German shepherd dogs, rottweilers) $\geq$2 years old. Body condition score was not reported (81).

Rupture of cranial cruciate ligament in the dog may also be associated with obesity. In one study, dogs with bilateral cranial cruciate ligament (CCL) rupture weighed more than dogs with unilateral CCL rupture; however, this was not statistically significant. Body condition score was not recorded in this study (82). In another study, obesity increased the risk of CCL rupture nearly 4 times when compared to ideal body weight dogs. The authors suggested this relationship between obesity and CCL rupture is due to the increased loading of the limbs and tension of the ligaments within the joints (83).

Perhaps not surprisingly, weight loss is one of the most effective treatment options for OA. Weight loss has been shown to improve locomotion in overweight dogs with OA (84–86). A significant reduction in lameness was seen in dogs with as little as 6.1% body weight loss (86). Although body weight and body condition score have not been as commonly implicated as a risk factor for development of orthopedic disease in cats (87), one study showed that overweight cats were 2.9 times more likely to present for evaluation of lameness than cats in optimal condition (24). The prevalence of feline hip dysplasia is significantly greater in Maine coon, Persian, and Himalayan cats, suggesting a possible link between body size and disease (88).

3.7.2 Neurologic disease

Dogs and cats with neurologic disease face similar locomotion issues as do animals with orthopedic disease. In dachshunds with intervertebral disc disease (IVDD), neither body weight nor BCS seems to be associated with risk of disease (89,90). However, other measurements of body size (e.g., longer T1-S1 distance, taller height at the withers, smaller pelvic circumference) were associated with severity of neurologic dysfunction (90). In a large group of dogs that underwent spinal decompression surgery for IVDD, there was a higher risk of development of postoperative discospondylitis in dogs that weighed >20 kg (91). Body condition was not assessed in this study. There was a very low incidence of discospondylitis (2.2%), and additional factors could have influenced these results (e.g., dog breed, length of anesthesia).

3.8 NEOPLASIA

Neoplasia is a broad disease group, with diverse findings regarding body composition and its relationship to disease prevalence and outcome. In a large prospective population-based study that followed 196 Leonbergers from birth to death, prevalence of primary bone tumors was assessed. Of the 196 dogs, 9 died from primary bone cancer. Those dogs were heavier during the growth period and early adult life, suggesting a possible influence of body composition on development of bone tumors (92). In a study of 325 dogs with splenic masses, the diagnosis of hemangiosarcoma was significantly less in dogs weighing ≤27.8 kg versus those weighing >27.8 kg (93). Overweight or obesity in dogs has been associated with a higher risk of development of mammary carcinoma, possibly due to tumor–adipocytes interactions and hormonal receptor-related tumor growth (94,95). Decreased adiponectin expression and increased macrophage numbers in overweight or obese dogs with mammary tumors were significantly correlated with factors related to a poor prognosis, such as high histologic grade and lymphatic invasion (94). When body composition is more closely assessed, there is a large range of BCS identified in dogs with cancer, likely dependent on the underlying neoplasm as well as comorbid diseases. In one study of 1777 dogs with cancer, the mean BCS was 5.3/9 (96). In another study, significantly more dogs were classified as being overweight (BCS ≥7/9%, 29%) versus underweight (BCS ≤3/9%, 4%) (97). Muscle loss (i.e., cachexia) was much more commonly observed in cats with various neoplasms than specifically a lower BCS (12).

In a study of cats with cancer, having a body weight >5 kg and/or BCS of ≥5/9 was significantly associated with better survival (12). In dogs diagnosed either with lymphoma or osteosarcoma, having a lower BCS at diagnosis was associated with a shorter survival time. Weight gain during treatment was associated with increased survival (98).

Before implementation of a purposeful weight loss plan in a cat or dog with obesity and neoplasia, a complete individual patient assessment should be performed, including cancer stage, clinical signs, and prognosis. One primary goal of weight loss in patients with neoplasia should be to improve quality of life. For example, in an obese dog that has undergone limb amputation for a primary bone tumor, weight loss may be imperative to improve the patient's mobility. In animals with neoplasms that are more prone to induce cachexia (e.g., gastrointestinal lymphoma), purposeful weight loss is likely only of benefit if the animal has comorbidities affected by overweight or obesity (e.g., significant respiratory compromise or osteoarthritis). Otherwise, it seems prudent to allow those animals to maintain a bit of excess weight, due to the obesity paradox phenomenon.

3.9 ANESTHETIC CONSIDERATIONS

Patients with excess body weight may present many difficulties for the anesthetist, including obesity-induced changes in organ system function, pharmacotherapeutic issues, and logistical challenges. Many published concerns and recommendations, including healthcare resource utilization, extended operative times, and increased risk of surgical site infection due to decreased subcutaneous oxygen tensions, are extrapolated from human evidence (99,100). Until more species-specific information is available, a conservative approach to anesthetic management of obese veterinary patients is warranted.

3.9.1 Obesity-induced alterations in physiology

3.9.1.1 RESPIRATORY PATHOPHYSIOLOGY

In the perioperative period, obese patients may desaturate quickly and display a tendency toward hypercapnia, sometimes severe (101). Obesity may complicate intubation because fat deposits in the pharyngeal cavity can make visualization of the airway difficult, especially in brachycephalic patients. Fat storage on the chest wall and abdomen affects functional respiratory mechanics, effectively stiffening the respiratory system. In addition, increased pulmonary blood volume and airway closure contribute to decreased respiratory compliance (102).

With increasing body mass, lung volumes are decreased, including tidal volumes and functional residual capacity (FRC). The FRC decreases exponentially and may approach residual volume (103,104). Breathing at low lung volumes reduces expiratory flow, increasing respiratory system resistance, and leads to airway closure and ventilation–perfusion mismatch. Obesity-associated increases in airway resistance and decreases in lung compliance increase the work of breathing. The walked distance during a 6-minute walk test (6MWT) was lower in obese dogs than lean subjects and weight loss was associated with improved walking distance (105). The authors of this study described the poor performance on the 6MWT as a marker of decreased quality of life in obese dogs and tentatively attributed this to obesity-associated respiratory dysfunction.

Tidal volumes are reduced and airflow limitations occur in obese cats (104,106). In obese dogs, reduced FRC and expiratory flow limitations have been documented during rebreathing-induced hyperpnea (103). No difference in inspiratory or expiratory flows was detected between obese and nonobese dogs at rest; however, in conscious upright obese humans the effect of obesity on airway function is small (107). The supine position (equivalent to dorsal recumbency in dogs and cats) increases expiratory flow limitations in obese humans. Airway hyperreactivity has been documented in obese beagles and may be governed by the systemic inflammatory state created by obesity; however, this finding was not replicated in obese cats (106,108).

Reduced respiratory compliance and lung volumes cause inequalities in distribution of ventilation and perfusion that can affect respiratory gas exchange. Hypoxemia at rest can be documented in obese humans, but a small study of 12 subjects did not confirm this finding in conscious obese dogs (108). In a clinical study of heavily sedated obese dogs, hypoxemia requiring oxygen supplementation was documented. The partial pressure of arterial oxygen (PaO_2) was improved and required oxygen supplementation decreased after weight loss, especially with decreased thoracic fat deposits as evidenced by dual-energy x-ray absorptiometry (109).

In order to maintain minute ventilation and avoid hypercapnia, respiratory rates are increased in obese humans and dogs (105,108,109). However, due to chronic reduction in respiratory compliance combined with increased airway resistance, ventilatory responses to carbon dioxide concentrations decline and obesity hypoventilation syndrome can develop. Supplementation of oxygen in the perioperative period can decrease ventilatory drive even further, and the anesthetist should be prepared to manually or mechanically support ventilation. Hypercapnia was not documented in 12 obese conscious dogs but the syndrome has not been specifically studied in companion animals (105).

Preoxygenation, recommended for all patients, is especially important for obese animals, as they may desaturate quickly upon induction of anesthesia. End-tidal expiratory carbon dioxide is a noninvasive and easily applied method for monitoring adequacy of ventilation during anesthesia. Manual or mechanical ventilation may be required in obese patients. Upper airway dysfunction may become especially relevant in the postanesthetic period. Obese patients should be monitored closely during recovery, and consideration should be given for oxygen supplementation during this time.

3.9.1.2 CARDIOVASCULAR PATHOPHYSIOLOGY

Experimentally induced obesity in dogs causes a sustained increase in sympathetic activity, increased resting heart rate, and decreased heart rate variability, eventually leading to systemic hypertension (110). Heart rate during rest and exercise are higher in obese dogs (BCS $\geq 8/9$) compared to lean (BCS 5/9) or merely overweight subjects (BCS 6–7/9) (105). Obesity has not been identified as a risk factor for systemic hypertension in a clinical population of dogs; however, a 5-point BCS was used in this study and an exact description of how the subjects were scored was not described (55). A separate study documented higher systolic arterial blood pressures (SAP) as measured by a Doppler device in obese (BCS $\geq 7/9$) versus lean (BCS $\leq 6/9$) dogs (111). The Mean $\pm$ SD for SAP for obese dogs was 153 ± 19 mm Hg, whereas it was 133 ± 20 mm Hg for lean dogs. Although these values were not significantly different, more obese dogs were classified as having moderate risk of end organ damage than lean dogs.

Various types of diastolic dysfunction have been identified in obese dogs, as evidenced by impaired relaxation and increased left ventricular filling pressures documented via echocardiography. Obese dogs displayed asymmetric concentric hypertrophy of the left ventricle without chamber dilation (111). The clinical significance of these changes and relevance to either myocardial or anesthetic outcomes are unclear; however, the possibility of systemic hypertension and/or diminished diastolic function should be recognized when developing perianesthetic management plans for obese dogs and cats.

3.9.1.3 OTHER ORGAN DYSFUNCTION

Of particular interest to the anesthetist is the possibility of feline DM with an almost fourfold increase in the likelihood of DM in obese versus lean cats (24). Management of blood glucose concentrations in the perioperative time period is required for diabetic cats and dogs; however, the required degree of blood glucose control to improve outcomes is unknown. Pain from osteoarthritis may be more prevalent in obese dogs and cats (112). Particular attention should be paid to limb placement and padding to avoid exacerbating painful joint disease. Specific perianesthetic management of other comorbidities, including collapsing trachea and various endocrine diseases, may be necessary and the obese patient should be screened carefully prior to anesthesia.

3.9.2 Pharmacological differences in obesity

Pharmacokinetic parameters may be affected by obesity. Pharmacokinetics concerns the absorption, distribution, metabolism, and elimination of drugs by the body.

3.9.2.1 DRUG ABSORPTION

Obesity may alter absorption of drugs in several ways. Subcutaneous blood flow is lower in obese subjects, and this may decrease or delay absorption of drugs administered via this route (113). Drugs intended for intramuscular administration may be inadvertently deposited subcutaneously due to the amount of fat tissue. For some drugs, this can drastically change absorption characteristics. For example, buprenorphine administered subcutaneously to cats is not reliably absorbed (and does not result in a detectable analgesic effect), whereas intramuscular and intravenous administration result in typical absorption and distribution characteristics as well as increased thermal thresholds (114).

3.9.2.2 DRUG DISTRIBUTION

Volume of distribution is a pharmacokinetic parameter used to determine the loading dose of a drug. It is the relationship at equilibrium between the amount of drug in the body and the plasma concentration and is dependent on the drug's physiochemical properties, tissue blood flow and protein binding. Changes in body composition can increase or decrease the volume of distribution, depending on whether the drug in question is lipophilic or hydrophilic. With developing obesity, lean body weight and fat weight increase but not in parallel, and the relationship between the two may even become inverted (i.e., the percentage of body fat may be greater than lean body weight)

(115). Most anesthetics and sedatives are lipophilic and may therefore experience a greater volume of distribution in obese patients. Tissue blood flow is also altered by obesity, with increases in blood volume and cardiac output due to higher metabolic demands of excess adipose tissue. In addition, cardiac dysfunction may alter tissue blood flow and drug distribution. These changes may result in an increased volume of distribution. Albumin binding of drugs appears to be unchanged in obesity, but uncertainty about alpha-1 acid glycoprotein binding of basic drugs exists (116).

Various recommendations have been made for alterations in bolus dosing of sedatives and anesthetics in obese human patients, including using ideal body weight for hydrophilic drugs, total body weight for lipophilic drugs, and an adjusted body weight (typically ideal body weight plus 20%–40%) for drugs that distribute to both adipose and lean tissue (117). Unfortunately, very little data supports these suggestions, as most pharmacokinetic studies are conducted in nonobese humans. Ideally, recommendations would be based on species-specific pharmacokinetic studies carried out in obese subjects. To date, only one study in dogs has investigated alterations in anesthetic drug requirements due to increased fat mass. This was a clinical study in which pharmacokinetic data were not collected. Based on total body weight, a lower dose of propofol (1.8 ± 0.4 mg/kg) was required in overweight and obese dogs versus normal weight controls (2.2 ± 0.5 mg/kg) following premedication with medetomidine and butorphanol (118). Lacking more rigorous evidence, the best approach is to carefully titrate initial bolus doses of injectable sedatives, analgesics, and anesthetics to effect.

3.9.2.3 DRUG METABOLISM AND ELIMINATION

Decline in drug plasma concentrations is termed "clearance" and is due to metabolic breakdown and elimination of the drug from the body. Clearance governs maintenance dosing of injectable drugs, whether by repeated bolus dosing or infusion. Plasma clearance is the sum of all organ clearances, including hepatic, renal, pulmonary, and other more typically minor routes. Changes in hepatic metabolism in obesity are variable with increases in obese humans and rats in the activity of cytochrome p450 (CYP) 2E1 enzyme, whereas clearance of drugs by CYP 3A4 is lower (119). No species-specific information is available for obese dogs or cats. As for initial loading doses, maintenance dosing of injectable agents should be carefully titrated to effect in obese animals.

3.10 CONCLUSION

Obesity can have a negative impact on life span, but the presence of excess body weight may actually improve survival times with cancer, heart failure, and CKD. Many endocrine, cardiovascular, respiratory, renal, urinary, orthopedic, neurologic, and neoplastic diseases will benefit from weight loss in overweight or obese cats and dogs, but consideration must be given to the level of weight loss required when the specific disease is associated with the obesity paradox. Patients with excess body weight also deserve additional considerations when undergoing anesthesia due to obesity-induced changes in organ system function, pharmacotherapeutic issues, and logistical challenges.

REFERENCES

1. Kealy RD, Lawler DF, Ballam JM et al. Effects of diet restriction on life span and age-related changes in dogs. *Journal of the American Veterinary Medical Association* 2002;220:1315–1320.
2. Richards SE, Wang Y, Claus SP et al. Metabolic phenotype modulation by caloric restriction in a lifelong dog study. *Journal of Proteome Research* 2013;12:3117–3127.
3. Greer KA, Canterberry SC, Murphy KE. Statistical analysis regarding the effects of height and weight on life span of the domestic dog. *Research in Veterinary Science* 2007;82:208–214.
4. Oga EA, Eseyin OR. The obesity paradox and heart failure: A systematic review of a decade of evidence. *J Obes* 2016;2016:9040248.
5. Carnethon MR, Rasmussen-Torvik LJ, Palaniappan L. The obesity paradox in diabetes. *Current Cardiology Reports* 2014;16:446.
6. Park J, Ahmadi S-F, Streja E et al. Obesity paradox in end-stage kidney disease patients. *Progress in Cardiovascular Diseases* 2014;56:415–425.
7. Kalantar-Zadeh K, Horwich TB, Oreopoulos A et al. Risk factor paradox in wasting diseases. *Current Opinion in Clinical Nutrition and Metabolic Care* 2007;10:433–442.
8. Kovesdy CP, Anderson JE, Kalantar-Zadeh K. Paradoxical association between body mass index and mortality in men with CKD not yet on dialysis. *American Journal of Kidney Diseases* 2007;49:581–591.
9. Fonarow GC, Srikanthan P, Costanzo MR et al. An obesity paradox in acute heart failure: Analysis of body mass index and inhospital mortality for 108,927 patients in the Acute Decompensated Heart Failure National Registry. *American Heart Journal* 2007;153:74–81.
10. Kapoor JR, Heidenreich PA. Obesity and survival in patients with heart failure and preserved systolic function: A U-shaped relationship. *American Heart Journal* 2010;159:75–80.
11. Johnson AP, Parlow JL, Whitehead M et al. Body mass index, outcomes, and mortality following cardiac surgery in Ontario, Canada. *Journal of the American Heart Association* 2015;4:e002140.
12. Baez JL, Michel KE, Sorenmo K et al. A prospective investigation of the prevalence and prognostic significance of weight loss and changes in body condition in feline cancer patients. *Journal of Feline Medicine and Surgery* 2007;9:411–417.
13. Slupe JL, Freeman LM, Rush JE. Association of body weight and body condition with survival in dogs with heart failure. *Journal of Veterinary Internal Medicine* 2008;22:561–565.
14. Finn E, Freeman LM, Rush JE et al. The relationship between body weight, body condition, and survival in cats with heart failure. *Journal of Veterinary Internal Medicine* 2010;24:1369–1374.
15. Parker VJ, Freeman LM. Association between body condition and survival in dogs with acquired chronic kidney disease. *Journal of Veterinary Internal Medicine* 2011;25:1306–1311.

16. Freeman LM, Lachaud MP, Matthews S et al. Evaluation of weight loss over time in cats with chronic kidney disease. *Journal of Veterinary Internal Medicine* 2016;30:1661–1666.
17. Morley JE, Thomas DR, Wilson MM. Cachexia: Pathophysiology and clinical relevance. *American Journal of Clinical Nutrition* 2006;83:735–743.
18. Mattin M, O'Neill D, Church D et al. An epidemiological study of diabetes mellitus in dogs attending first opinion practice in the UK. *The Veterinary Record* 2014;174:349.
19. Raffan E, Dennis RJ, O'Donovan CJ et al. A deletion in the canine POMC gene is associated with weight and appetite in obesity-prone Labrador retriever dogs. *Cell Metabolism* 2016;23:893–900.
20. Davison LJ, Holder A, Catchpole B et al. The canine POMC gene, obesity in Labrador retrievers and susceptibility to diabetes mellitus. *Journal of Veterinary Internal Medicine* 2017;31:343–348.
21. Verkest KR, Fleeman LM, Morton JM et al. Compensation for obesity-induced insulin resistance in dogs: Assessment of the effects of leptin, adiponectin, and glucagon-like peptide-1 using path analysis. *Domestic Animal Endocrinology* 2011;41:24–34.
22. Bailhache E, Nguyen P, Krempf M et al. Lipoproteins abnormalities in obese insulin-resistant dogs. *Metabolism* 2003;52:559–564.
23. German AJ, Hervera M, Hunter L et al. Improvement in insulin resistance and reduction in plasma inflammatory adipokines after weight loss in obese dogs. *Domestic Animal Endocrinology* 2009;37:214–226.
24. Scarlett JM, Donoghue S. Associations between body condition and disease in cats. *Journal of the American Veterinary Medical Association* 1998;212:1725–1731.
25. Hoenig M, Pach N, Thomaseth K et al. Cats differ from other species in their cytokine and antioxidant enzyme response when developing obesity. *Obesity (Silver Spring)* 2013;21:E407–E414.
26. Hoenig M, Thomaseth K, Waldron M et al. Insulin sensitivity, fat distribution, and adipocytokine response to different diets in lean and obese cats before and after weight loss. *American Journal of Physiology: Regulatory, Integrative and Comparative Physiology* 2007;292:R227–R234.
27. Forcada Y, Holder A, Church DB et al. A polymorphism in the melanocortin 4 receptor gene (MC4R:c.92C>T) is associated with diabetes mellitus in overweight domestic shorthaired cats. *Journal of Veterinary Internal Medicine* 2014;28:458–464.
28. Ishioka K, Omachi A, Sasaki N et al. Feline adiponectin: Molecular structures and plasma concentrations in obese cats. *Journal of Veterinary Medical Science* 2009;71:189–194.
29. Bjornvad CR, Rand JS, Tan HY et al. Obesity and sex influence insulin resistance and total and multimer adiponectin levels in adult neutered domestic shorthair client-owned cats. *Domestic Animal Endocrinology* 2014;47:55–64.

30. Zapata RC, Meachem MD, Cardoso NC et al. Differential circulating concentrations of adipokines, glucagon and adropin in a clinical population of lean, overweight and diabetic cats. *BMC Veterinary Research* 2017;13:85.

31. Öhlund M, Egenvall A, Fall T et al. Environmental risk factors for diabetes mellitus in cats. *Journal of Veterinary Internal Medicine* 2017;31:29–35.

32. Rowe E, Browne W, Casey R et al. Risk factors identified for owner-reported feline obesity at around one year of age: Dry diet and indoor lifestyle. *Preventive Veterinary Medicine* 2015;121:273–281.

33. Plantinga EA, Bosch G, Hendriks WH. Estimation of the dietary nutrient profile of free-roaming feral cats: Possible implications for nutrition of domestic cats. *British Journal of Nutrition* 2011;106:S35–S48.

34. Verbrugghe A, Hesta M. Cats and carbohydrates: The carnivore fantasy? *Vet Sci* 2017;4:E55.

35. Bennett N, Greco DS, Peterson ME et al. Comparison of a low carbohydrate-low fiber diet and a moderate carbohydrate-high fiber diet in the management of feline diabetes mellitus. *Journal of Feline Medicine and Surgery* 2006;8:73–84.

36. Mazzaferro EM, Greco DS, Turner AS et al. Treatment of feline diabetes mellitus using an alpha-glucosidase inhibitor and a low-carbohydrate diet. *Journal of Feline Medicine and Surgery* 2003;5:183–189.

37. Frank G, Anderson W, Pazak H et al. Use of a high-protein diet in the management of feline diabetes mellitus. *Veterinary Therapeutics: Research in Applied Veterinary Medicine* 2001;2:238–246.

38. Cho K-D, Paek J, Kang J-H et al. Serum adipokine concentrations in dogs with naturally occurring pituitary-dependent hyperadrenocorticism. *Journal of Veterinary Internal Medicine* 2014;28:429–436.

39. Katagiri H, Yamada T, Oka Y. Adiposity and cardiovascular disorders: Disturbance of the regulatory system consisting of humoral and neuronal signals. *Circulation Research* 2007;101:27–39.

40. Cabrera Blatter MF, del Prado B, Miceli DD et al. Interleukin-6 and insulin increase and nitric oxide and adiponectin decrease in blind dogs with pituitary-dependent hyperadrenocorticism. *Research in Veterinary Science* 2012;93:1195–1202.

41. Greco DS, Rosychuk RA, Ogilvie GK et al. The effect of levothyroxine treatment on resting energy expenditure of hypothyroid dogs. *Journal of Veterinary Internal Medicine* 1998;12:7–10.

42. Chikamune T, Katamoto H, Ohashi F et al. Serum lipid and lipoprotein concentrations in obese dogs. *Journal of Veterinary Medical Science* 1995;57:595–598.

43. Jeusette IC, Lhoest ET, Istasse LP et al. Influence of obesity on plasma lipid and lipoprotein concentrations in dogs. *American Journal of Veterinary Research* 2005;66:81–86.

44. Hoenig M, Wilkins C, Holson JC et al. Effects of obesity on lipid profiles in neutered male and female cats. *American Journal of Veterinary Research* 2003;64:299–303.

45. Hoenig M, Traas AM, Schaeffer DJ. Evaluation of routine hematology profile results and fructosamine, thyroxine, insulin, and proinsulin concentrations in lean, overweight, obese, and diabetic cats. *Journal of the American Veterinary Medical Association* 2013;243:1302–1309.

46. Diez M, Michaux C, Jeusette I et al. Evolution of blood parameters during weight loss in experimental obese Beagle dogs. *Journal of Animal Physiology and Animal Nutrition* 2004;88:166–171.

47. Peña C, Suarez L, Bautista-Castaño I et al. Effects of low-fat high-fibre diet and mitratapide on body weight reduction, blood pressure and metabolic parameters in obese dogs. *Journal of Veterinary Medical Science* 2014;76:1305–1308.

48. Xenoulis PG, Steiner JM. Canine hyperlipidaemia. *Journal of Small Animal Practice* 2015;56:595–605.

49. Jordan E, Kley S, Le N-A et al. Dyslipidemia in obese cats. *Domestic Animal Endocrinology* 2008;35:290–299.

50. Nishii N, Maeda H, Murahata Y et al. Experimental hyperlipemia induces insulin resistance in cats. *Journal of Veterinary Medical Science* 2012;74:267–269.

51. Fonfara S, Hetzel U, Tew SR et al. Leptin expression in dogs with cardiac disease and congestive heart failure. *Journal of Veterinary Internal Medicine* 2011;25:1017–1024.

52. Jahangir E, De Schutter A, Lavie CJ. The relationship between obesity and coronary artery disease. *Translational Research: The Journal of Laboratory and Clinical Medicine* 2014;164:336–344.

53. Rocchini AP, Moorehead C, Wentz E et al. Obesity-induced hypertension in the dog. *Hypertension* 1987;9:II164–II168.

54. Granger JP, West D, Scott J. Abnormal pressure natriuresis in the dog model of obesity-induced hypertension. *Hypertension* 1994;23:I8–I11.

55. Pérez-Sánchez AP, Del-Angel-Caraza J, Quijano-Hernández IA et al. Obesity-hypertension and its relation to other diseases in dogs. *Veterinary Research Communications* 2015;39:45–51.

56. Bodey AR, Michell AR. Epidemiological study of blood pressure in domestic dogs. *Journal of Small Animal Practice* 1996;37:116–125.

57. Montoya JA, Morris PJ, Bautista I et al. Hypertension: A risk factor associated with weight status in dogs. *Journal of Nutrition* 2006;136:2011S–2013S.

58. Rubin JA, Holt DE, Reetz JA et al. Signalment, clinical presentation, concurrent diseases, and diagnostic findings in 28 dogs with dynamic pharyngeal collapse (2008–2013). *Journal of Veterinary Internal Medicine* 2015;29:815–821.

59. Tinga S, Thieman Mankin KM, Peycke LE et al. Comparison of outcome after use of extra-luminal rings and intra-luminal stents for treatment of tracheal collapse in dogs. *Veterinary Surgery* 2015;44:858–865.

60. Maggiore AD. Tracheal and airway collapse in dogs. *The Veterinary Clinics of North America: Small Animal Practice* 2014;44:117–127.

61. Greene JP, Lefebvre SL, Wang M et al. Risk factors associated with the development of chronic kidney disease in cats evaluated at primary care veterinary hospitals. *Journal of the American Veterinary Medical Association* 2014;244:320–327.

62. Henegar JR, Bigler SA, Henegar LK et al. Functional and structural changes in the kidney in the early stages of obesity. *Journal of the American Society of Nephrology* 2001;12:1211–1217.

63. Tvarijonaviciute A, Ceron JJ, Holden SL et al. Effect of weight loss in obese dogs on indicators of renal function or disease. *Journal of Veterinary Internal Medicine* 2013;27:31–38.

64. Tefft KM, Shaw DH, Ihle SL et al. Association between excess body weight and urine protein concentration in healthy dogs. *Veterinary Clinical Pathology* 2014;43:255–260.

65. Cameron ME, Casey RA, Bradshaw JW et al. A study of environmental and behavioural factors that may be associated with feline idiopathic cystitis. *Journal of Small Animal Practice* 2004;45:144–147.

66. Defauw PAM, Van de Maele I, Duchateau L et al. Risk factors and clinical presentation of cats with feline idiopathic cystitis. *Journal of Feline Medicine and Surgery* 2011;13:967–975.

67. Lund HS, Krontveit RI, Halvorsen I et al. Evaluation of urinalyses from untreated adult cats with lower urinary tract disease and healthy control cats: Predictive abilities and clinical relevance. *Journal of Feline Medicine and Surgery* 2013;15:1086–1097.

68. Jones BR, Sanson RL, Morris RS. Elucidating the risk factors of feline lower urinary tract disease. *New Zealand Veterinary Journal* 1997;45:100–108.

69. Lekcharoensuk C, Osborne CA, Lulich JP. Epidemiologic study of risk factors for lower urinary tract diseases in cats. *Journal of the American Veterinary Medical Association* 2001;218:1429–1435.

70. Segev G, Livne H, Ranen E et al. Urethral obstruction in cats: Predisposing factors, clinical, clinicopathological characteristics and prognosis. *Journal of Feline Medicine and Surgery* 2011;13:101–108.

71. Kennedy SM, Lulich JP, Ritt MG et al. Comparison of body condition score and urinalysis variables between dogs with and without calcium oxalate uroliths. *Journal of the American Veterinary Medical Association* 2016;249:1274–1280.

72. Subak LL, Richter HE, Hunskaar S. Obesity and urinary incontinence: Epidemiology and clinical research update. *Journal of Urology* 2009;182:S2–S7.

73. Wynn SG, Witzel AL, Bartges JW et al. Prevalence of asymptomatic urinary tract infections in morbidly obese dogs. *PeerJ* 2016;4:e1711.

74. Kapoor M, Martel-Pelletier J, Lajeunesse D et al. Role of proinflammatory cytokines in the pathophysiology of osteoarthritis. *Nature Reviews: Rheumatology* 2011;7:33–42.

75. Backus R, Wara A. Development of obesity: Mechanisms and physiology. *The Veterinary Clinics of North America: Small Animal Practice* 2016;46:773–784.

76. Frank L, Mann S, Levine CB et al. Increasing body condition score is positively associated interleukin-6 and monocyte chemoattractant protein-1 in Labrador retrievers. *Veterinary Immunology and Immunopathology* 2015;167:104–109.

77. Collins KH, Paul HA, Reimer RA et al. Relationship between inflammation, the gut microbiota, and metabolic osteoarthritis development: Studies in a rat model. *Osteoarthritis and Cartilage* 2015;23:1989–1998.

78. Edney AT, Smith PM. Study of obesity in dogs visiting veterinary practices in the United Kingdom. *The Veterinary Record* 1986;118:391–396.

79. Huck JL, Biery DN, Lawler DF et al. A longitudinal study of the influence of lifetime food restriction on development of osteoarthritis in the canine elbow. *Veterinary Surgery* 2009;38:192–198.

80. Smith GK, Paster ER, Powers MY et al. Lifelong diet restriction and radiographic evidence of osteoarthritis of the hip joint in dogs. *Journal of the American Veterinary Medical Association* 2006;229:690–693.

81. Smith GK, Mayhew PD, Kapatkin AS et al. Evaluation of risk factors for degenerative joint disease associated with hip dysplasia in German Shepherd Dogs, Golden Retrievers, Labrador Retrievers, and Rottweilers. *Journal of the American Veterinary Medical Association* 2001;219:1719–1724.

82. Grierson J, Asher L, Grainger K. An investigation into risk factors for bilateral canine cruciate ligament rupture. *Veterinary and Comparative Orthopaedics and Traumatology* 2011;24:192–196.

83. Adams P, Bolus R, Middleton S et al. Influence of signalment on developing cranial cruciate rupture in dogs in the UK. *Journal of Small Animal Practice* 2011;52:347–352.

84. Impellizeri JA, Tetrick MA, Muir P. Effect of weight reduction on clinical signs of lameness in dogs with hip osteoarthritis. *Journal of the American Veterinary Medical Association* 2000;216:1089–1091.

85. Mlacnik E, Bockstahler BA, Müller M et al. Effects of caloric restriction and a moderate or intense physiotherapy program for treatment of lameness in overweight dogs with osteoarthritis. *Journal of the American Veterinary Medical Association* 2006;229:1756–1760.

86. Marshall WG, Hazewinkel HAW, Mullen D et al. The effect of weight loss on lameness in obese dogs with osteoarthritis. *Veterinary Research Communications* 2010;34:241–253.

87. Bennett D, Zainal Ariffin SM, Johnston P. Osteoarthritis in the cat: 1. How common is it and how easy to recognise? *Journal of Feline Medicine and Surgery* 2012;14:65–75.

88. Keller GG, Reed AL, Lattimer JC et al. Hip dysplasia: A feline population study. *Veterinary Radiology & Ultrasound* 1999;40:460–464.

89. Jensen VF, Ersbøll AK. Mechanical factors affecting the occurrence of intervertebral disc calcification in the dachshund – A population study. *Journal of Veterinary Medicine. A, Physiology, Pathology, Clinical Medicine* 2000;47:283–296.

90. Levine JM, Levine GJ, Kerwin SC et al. Association between various physical factors and acute thoracolumbar intervertebral disk extrusion or protrusion in Dachshunds. *Journal of the American Veterinary Medical Association* 2006;229:370–375.

91. Canal S, Contiero B, Balducci F et al. Risk factors for diskospondylitis in dogs after spinal decompression surgery for intervertebral disk herniation. *Journal of the American Veterinary Medical Association* 2016;248:1383–1390.

92. Anfinsen KP, Grotmol T, Bruland OS et al. Primary bone cancer in Leonbergers may be associated with a higher bodyweight during adolescence. *Preventive Veterinary Medicine* 2015;119:48–53.

93. Sherwood JM, Haynes AM, Klocke E et al. Occurrence and clinicopathologic features of splenic neoplasia based on body weight: 325 dogs (2003–2013). *Journal of the American Animal Hospital Association* 2016;52:220–226.

94. Lim HY, Im KS, Kim NH et al. Obesity, expression of adipocytokines, and macrophage infiltration in canine mammary tumors. *Veterinary Journal* 2015;203:326–331.

95. Lim H-Y, Im K-S, Kim N-H et al. Effects of obesity and obesity-related molecules on canine mammary gland tumors. *Veterinary Pathology* 2015;52:1045–1051.

96. Weeth LP, Fascetti AJ, Kass PH et al. Prevalence of obese dogs in a population of dogs with cancer. *American Journal of Veterinary Research* 2007;68:389–398.

97. Michel KE, Sorenmo K, Shofer FS. Evaluation of body condition and weight loss in dogs presented to a veterinary oncology service. *Journal of Veterinary Internal Medicine* 2004;18:692–695.

98. Romano FR, Heinze CR, Barber LG et al. Association between body condition score and cancer prognosis in dogs with lymphoma and osteosarcoma. *Journal of Veterinary Internal Medicine* 2016;30:1179–1186.

99. Kadry B, Press CD, Alosh H et al. Obesity increases operating room times in patients undergoing primary hip arthroplasty: A retrospective cohort analysis. *PeerJ* 2014;2:e530.

100. Kabon B, Nagele A, Reddy D et al. Obesity decreases perioperative tissue oxygenation. *Anesthesiology* 2004;100:274–280.

101. Hedenstierna G, Santesson J. Breathing mechanics, dead space and gas exchange in the extremely obese, breathing spontaneously and during anaesthesia with intermittent positive pressure ventilation. *Acta Anaesthesiologica Scandinavica* 1976;20:248–254.

102. Salome CM, King GG, Berend N. Physiology of obesity and effects on lung function. *Journal of Applied Physiology* 2010;108:206–211.

103. Jones RL, Nzekwu MM. The effects of body mass index on lung volumes. *Chest* 2006;130:827–833.

104. Bach JF, Rozanski EA, Bedenice D et al. Association of expiratory airway dysfunction with marked obesity in healthy adult dogs. *American Journal of Veterinary Research* 2007;68:670–675.

105. Manens J, Ricci R, Damoiseaux C et al. Effect of body weight loss on cardiopulmonary function assessed by 6-minute walk test and arterial blood gas analysis in obese dogs. *Journal of Veterinary Internal Medicine* 2014;28:371–378.
106. García-Guasch L, Caro-Vadillo A, Manubens-Grau J et al. Pulmonary function in obese vs non-obese cats. *Journal of Feline Medicine and Surgery* 2015;17:494–499.
107. Ferretti A, Giampiccolo P, Cavalli A et al. Expiratory flow limitation and orthopnea in massively obese subjects. *Chest* 2001;119:1401–1408.
108. Manens J, Bolognin M, Bernaerts F et al. Effects of obesity on lung function and airway reactivity in healthy dogs. *Veterinary Journal* 2012;193:217–221.
109. Mosing M, German AJ, Holden SL et al. Oxygenation and ventilation characteristics in obese sedated dogs before and after weight loss: A clinical trial. *Veterinary Journal* 2013;198:367–371.
110. Iliescu R, Tudorancea I, Irwin ED et al. Chronic baroreflex activation restores spontaneous baroreflex control and variability of heart rate in obesity-induced hypertension. *American Journal of Physiology: Heart and Circulatory Physiology* 2013;305:H1080–H1088.
111. Mehlman E, Bright JM, Jeckel K et al. Echocardiographic evidence of left ventricular hypertrophy in obese dogs. *Journal of Veterinary Internal Medicine* 2013;27:62–68.
112. Marshall W, Bockstahler B, Hulse D et al. A review of osteoarthritis and obesity: Current understanding of the relationship and benefit of obesity treatment and prevention in the dog. *Veterinary and Comparative Orthopaedics and Traumatology* 2009;22:339–345.
113. Summers LK, Samra JS, Humphreys SM et al. Subcutaneous abdominal adipose tissue blood flow: Variation within and between subjects and relationship to obesity. *Clinical Science (London)* 1996;91:679–683.
114. Steagall PV, Pelligand L, Giordano T et al. Pharmacokinetic and pharmacodynamic modelling of intravenous, intramuscular and subcutaneous buprenorphine in conscious cats. *Veterinary Anaesthesia and Analgesia* 2013;40:83–95.
115. Ingrande J, Lemmens HJ. Dose adjustment of anaesthetics in the morbidly obese. *British Journal of Anaesthesia* 2010;105:i16–i23.
116. Hanley MJ, Abernethy DR, Greenblatt DJ. Effect of obesity on the pharmacokinetics of drugs in humans. *Clinical Pharmacokinetics* 2010;49:71–87.
117. Cheymol G. Effects of obesity on pharmacokinetics implications for drug therapy. *Clinical Pharmacokinetics* 2000;39:215–231.
118. Boveri S, Brearley JC, Dugdale AH. The effect of body condition on propofol requirement in dogs. *Veterinary Anaesthesia and Analgesia* 2013;40:449–454.
119. Brill MJ, Diepstraten J, van Rongen A et al. Impact of obesity on drug metabolism and elimination in adults and children. *Clinical Pharmacokinetics* 2012;51:277–304.

4

Evaluation of body composition to diagnose obesity

CHARLOTTE REINHARD BJØRNVAD AND
LENE ELISABETH BUELUND

4.1 INTRODUCTION

A failure to recognize an overweight/obese status is likely a main contributing factor to obesity being the main nutritional disorder in dogs and cats. Owners are often unable to correctly assess the degree of obesity in their pet, and especially in overweight and obese pets, they tend to underestimate the body condition score (BCS) (1–5). This highlights the veterinarian's role in identifying pets as overweight/obese to initiate appropriate preventative and treatment interventions.

However, in both large referral and smaller private veterinary clinics there is generally a failure in recording the patient's BCS and even if recorded, actions in relation to a BCS below or above normal are often lacking (6–9). In response to this, the World Small Animal Veterinary Association (WSAVA) introduced "nutritional assessment" as the fifth vital sign in 2011 (10). For all pets visiting a veterinarian, the clinician should always perform a nutritional assessment including body condition scoring as well as measure body temperature, pulse rate, respiration rate, and conduct pain assessment. Additionally, the American Animal Hospital Association (AAHA) weight management guidelines from 2014 advises veterinarians to "monitor weight trends and proactively address weight gain early at any BCS above the ideal" both during growth, post gonadectomy, and at following yearly examinations (11). Currently, there are several methods available for evaluating body composition in pets; some are more objective but expensive and require specialized equipment, whereas some are less expensive and easier to implement in a clinical practice setting. To appropriately use the different tools, it is important to understand their strengths and limitations, and be aware of the accuracy (the ability to provide correct measurements reflecting the true or absolute value) and precision (the ability to provide reliable and consistent measurements) relating to each method. In the following we will describe and discuss the most commonly used or best evaluated methodologies for ante- and postmortem evaluation of body composition in dogs and cats.

4.2 CARCASS ANALYSIS OF BODY COMPOSITION

Carcass analysis is a chemical analysis of body constituents and it is considered the gold standard for evaluating body composition across species (12). The method includes dissection of all tissues followed by grounding/homogenization of the tissues. Water content is assessed by drying known quantities of tissue in an oven or by freeze-drying (lyophilizing) and measuring the weight differences before and after the drying. Fat content is estimated by using organic solvents, and mineral content is determined by burning all organic matter in a sample (12,13). For small subjects where the whole body can be analyzed and when it can be performed right after euthanasia, it is a very accurate methodology. However, if the carcass is frozen prior to analysis, water evaporation may affect the measurement, and with larger subjects only smaller subsamples that may not completely reflect the total composition are analyzed (13,14). In addition, when a whole carcass is being processed, content of the gastrointestinal (GI) tract may affect results. These issues can, however, be addressed by estimating water loss by weighing the animal before and after freezing, and by fasting, evisceration, or emptying the gut prior to analysis (13). Because this methodology can only be applied following euthanasia of the animal, it is mainly useful in research settings and in validating other methods and not in veterinary practice.

Most other techniques for evaluating body composition are based on indirect methods that use the model of the body being at least two chemically distinct compartments, often including the fat and the fat-free mass (FFM) (14). However, the measured compartments differ in methodologies used, as illustrated in Table 4.1 (15).

Table 4.1 Body composition terms and their relation to common body composition measurement methods used for dogs and cats

Term	Explanation	Measurement methods
Body fat mass	Quantity of triglyceride fat in the body	Carcass analysis Dual energy x-ray absorptiometry (Bioelectrical impedance analysis) Anthropometry Body condition scoring
Adipose tissue mass	Fat ($\sim$83%) plus supporting cellular and extracellular structures (consisting of $\sim$2% protein and $\sim$15% water)	Computed tomography Magnetic resonance imaging
Lean body mass	Nonadipose tissue body mass (including bone mineral)	D_2O Computed tomography Magnetic resonance imaging
Fat-free mass	Lean body mass plus nonfat components of adipose tissue	Carcass analysis Bioelectrical impedance analysis (Dual energy x-ray absorptiometry)
Body cell mass	Cellular components of the body	D_2O
Extracellular solids (ECS)	Total body bone mineral (skeleton $\sim$85% of ECS) + fascia, cartilage and so forth ($\sim$15% of ECS)	Carcass analysis Dual energy x-ray absorptiometry

Source: Modified from Jensen MD. *Journal of the American Dietetic Association* 1992;92(4):454–60.

Note: When method is in parentheses, the value is calculated based on other measurements obtained with the method.

4.3 IMAGING MODALITIES TO ASSESS BODY COMPOSITION

4.3.1 Dual energy x-ray absorptiometry (DEXA)

Initially developed and used for evaluation of bone mineral content in humans, the dual energy x-ray absorptiometry (DEXA) method has advanced into a useful tool for body composition assessment (16,17). In veterinary research DEXA has proven useful especially for assessment of bone mineral content and body composition, providing measurements of bone mass, fat mass, and lean soft tissue mass (18) (Figure 4.1). The term "lean body mass" is often used interchangeably with "lean soft tissue mass" in connection to DEXA. However, by definition, lean body mass includes bone minerals that are measured separately with DEXA (19). Clear definitions of different body compartments are lacking, which may lead to possible errors in data reporting due to overlap or omission of specific compartments. Clarifications of terms and definitions have been proposed (19–21), where it is suggested that lean body mass is synonymous with fat-free mass as illustrated in Figure 4.1.

The physical principle behind DEXA is the measuring of attenuation of two x-ray beams, at low and high photon energy levels, after they have passed

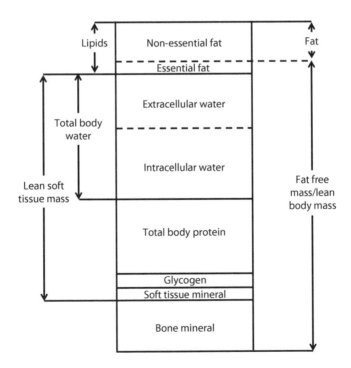

Figure 4.1 Body composition measurements and terms. Discrepancies exist concerning the definition of lean body mass. In this figure, lean body mass is defined as equivalent to fat-free mass. (Adapted from Heymsfield SB et al. *Annual Review of Nutrition* 1997;17:527–58.)

through the body. By using different algorithms, the DEXA scanner can quantitate the different types of tissues for each pixel resulting in estimates of total mass, bone mineral content, fat, and lean soft tissue mass (15,17,22). The radiation burden during a DEXA scan is low (17). The physical concept of DEXA and body composition has been described in detail in the review of Pietrobelli et al. (20).

DEXA systems are produced by a limited number of manufacturers, and although based on the same physical principles, they differ regarding the generation of the high- and low-energy x-ray beams, the x-ray detectors, the imaging geometry, the calibration methodology, and software algorithms (22). The systems come with different software packages including analysis for small animals, and pediatric and adult humans. Interdevice differences are therefore inevitable and comparison of results for estimates of bone mineral content and body composition should be performed with caution (23–25).

Validation of DEXA has been conducted by comparison to carcass chemical analysis in several species (12,26–34). DEXA estimates of total mass and scale measurements have consistently shown high correlation (12,28–33,35). Investigation of canine body composition has revealed no significant difference between percentage body fat or percentage fat-free mass as estimated by DEXA and from chemical analysis (26). However, a significant difference has been observed in bone mineral content between DEXA measurement and ash percentage (26). Within the study of Speakman et al., strong correlation between estimates of total body mass ($r^2 = 1.00$), fat-free mass ($r^2 = 0.998$), and fat mass ($r^2 = 0.964$) was found in both cats and dogs. Mean error for fat-free mass component was 2.64% and 2.04% for fat tissue. However, fat-free mass differences ranged from −2.64% underestimation to 13.22% overestimation, while for fat mass it varied from −20.7% underestimation to 31.5% overestimation, presumably related to the muscular hydration status (12). Studies using pigs and piglets within the weight range of cats and dogs have also shown high correlation between DEXA measurements and chemical analysis, though substantial differences in absolute fat mass have been observed (27–29,31–33). These differences have been suggested to reflect differences between the different instrument manufacturers and analyzing software (24,32), but also incomplete homogenization of the carcasses for chemical analysis has been considered (27). Newer instruments, refinement of software, and specific calibration factors have improved the accuracy further (29,36,37). Validation studies in feline, canine, and porcine species have found that the DEXA technique provides good precision in measuring body compartments (26–28,32,38–40). However, consistently the determination of fat mass has the poorest coefficient of variation (CV) reported, approaching 6% as shown in cats in one study (38).

DEXA is often considered the second best after carcass analysis for body composition analysis of cats and dogs. It has been used for determining intra- and interbreed variation in body composition in a variety of dog breeds (12,26), for estimation of body composition and weight changes in cats and dogs (40–44), and for validation of other methods for assessment of body composition such as bioimpedance, body fat index systems, and body condition scores (45–52).

4.3.2 Computer tomography (CT)

As with DEXA, computer tomography (CT) is based on x-ray technology, however, with a more pronounced radiation burden to follow. Within CT scans measurement of the attenuation of x-rays are obtained from a large number of angles. The subsequent CT reconstruction converts the raw acquired data to series of CT images, each image built up by volume elements, or voxels. The average linear attenuation coefficient in each voxel is expressed using the Hounsfield unit (HU) scale, where the value 0 HU corresponds to the linear attenuation coefficient of water and −1000 HU corresponds to the linear attenuation coefficient of air. As the physical density is one of the main determinants of attenuation, tissues such as adipose tissue and soft tissue, each possessing unique tissue densities, can be discriminated by the HU number. Using the detailed CT images and voxel measurements it is possible not only to determine lean and adipose tissue, but also tissue distribution, for example, estimating visceral and subcutaneous fat compartments (53).

Even though the number of CT scanners in veterinary medicine is increasing, only a limited number of body compositional studies within companion animals are available and validation studies are limited. Ishioka et al. validated CT scans of seven beagles against the deuterium oxide (D_2O) dilution technique and proposed a range from −105 to −135 HU as dog-specific adipose tissue ranges, and sampling at the level of the third lumbar vertebra (L3; $r^2 = 0.96$) was valuable for assessing body fat content (54). The attenuation range for feline adipose tissue has been determined to be between −106 and –156 HU with L3 and L5 as optimal sampling sites for the entire abdominal volume (55). To overcome the need of tissue specific HU ranges such as the ranges suggested by Ishioka et al. and Lee et al. (54,55), investigating the frequency distribution of voxels by Hounsfield unit values has been conducted. Here it was possible to establish an adipose tissue percentage in cats correlating with the body fat percentages obtained with DEXA (56). CT has also been used for assessing visceral and subcutaneous fat mass in relation to distribution of weight gain and body compositional changes related to neutering and different biomarkers in metabolic diseases (54,57,58).

4.3.3 Magnetic resonance imaging (MRI)

In contrast to DEXA and CT, magnetic resonance imaging (MRI) does not use ionizing radiation such as x-rays. Instead MRI is based on the interaction between a generated magnetic field and protons, that is, hydrogen nuclei, which are abundant in biological tissue (53).

MRI produces tomographic images. As different types of tissue, such as adipose tissue, brain parenchyma, and so forth have different local magnetic properties, MRI provides high contrast images with high sensitivity to anatomical variation (53).

Only a limited number of publications are available concerning MRI and body composition in companion animals. Assessment of obesity by MRI has been conducted in cats (59) and whole-body fat–water MRI (FWMRI) have been successfully applied in dogs before and after weight gain in combination with semiautomatic image analysis (60). FWMRI estimates of total mass were in accordance with scale weight ($r^2 = 0.867$), and following weight gain, significant increases in visceral, subcutaneous, and total adipose tissue were shown. FWMRI was a precise method for measurement of total adipose tissue, visceral tissue, lean tissue, and cortical bone with CV in the range of 0.2%–3.1% (60).

Using a newer technique called quantitative magnetic resonance (QMR), body composition measurements have been validated against D_2O and DEXA in dogs and cats showing that QMR is a promising tool for body composition measurements, though significant underestimation of total body weight, lean body mass, and fat mass was found in dogs when compared to D_2O (61). In cats a significant underestimation was only found for fat mass when compared to D_2O (62). Apart from being spared from ionizing radiation, the QMR method can be performed in unsedated animals. By implementing appropriate correction equations, QMR is promising as a tool for providing accurate assessment of body composition (61,62).

Imaging modalities provide noninvasive measurements that are objective and reproducible. Specialized equipment such as DEXA scanners, CT, and MRI scanners, are limited to use at larger veterinary centers and university hospitals. In addition, general anesthesia or sedation is often necessary, and some modalities involve a radiation burden on both animal and staff (Figure 4.2).

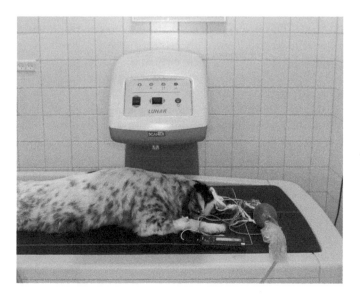

Figure 4.2 Photographic view of a dual energy x-ray absorptiometry scan on an anesthetized dog in ventral recumbency. During the scan, the large scanning arm passes over the patient. Pulse oximetry equipment is present on the scan table. (Courtesy of A.D. Vitger.)

4.4 NONIMAGING-BASED MODALITIES TO ASSESS BODY COMPOSITION

4.4.1 Deuterium oxide dilution technique

The deuterium oxide (D_2O) dilution technique is based on the fact that body water is predominantly associated with nonfat tissue; thus, total body water measurement provides an indirect measure of fat-free mass (13). Deuterium oxide is a stable, nontoxic tracer that is freely exchangeable with water. Following intravenous administration of a known quantity of D_2O, it will, given time, distribute uniformly throughout the different body water pools. When equilibrium is reached, total body water can be assessed by measuring the degree of dilution of the tracer in a blood sample (13,63). Based on the assumption that fat-free mass contains 73.2% water, body fat percentage (BF%) can be calculated using the following formula: BF% = 100 – percent total body water/0.732 (13,46,63). It has been proposed that a possible loss of isotopes through pulmonary respiration and urine is inevitable and could affect the results. However, in a study in dogs, urinary loss was determined to be insignificant (13,63). Compared with carcass analysis, D_2O overestimated amount of body water by 21.8%, which was evaluated as relatively high, and several equations could not be validated due to nonparametric data. However, correlation based on proposed equations was good; percent body water ($r^2 = 0.96$), percent body fat ($r^2 = 0.96$), percent nitrogen ($r^2 = 0.77$), and percent ash ($r^2 = 0.64$) (13). Studies in dogs have revealed an overestimation of body fat by DEXA scans in comparison to D_2O around 13%–15.8%. Though having lack of absolute agreement, the two methods showed a good correlation ($r^2 = 0.78$) (35,46). Taking the possible systematic underestimation of BF% into account, most studies have shown an excellent relative agreement between the D_2O dilution technique, carcass analyses, and DEXA in both dogs and cats (35,46,61–63). Time for isotope equilibration, however, affects results and should be standardized (13,64).

The D_2O dilution technique is a safe and noninvasive method for providing quantitative measures for body composition in dogs and cats. It is, however, expensive, requires hospitalization until equilibrium is reached, and therefore is primarily used for research.

4.4.2 Bioimpedance

Bioimpedance (BIA) measures the resistance to an electrical signal through the water contained in muscle and fat tissues. High muscle and low fat mass result in a higher body water content that facilitates the flow of an electrical current through the body. With more fat present, the resistance increases and the electrical flow declines (65,66). The methodology is described as a safe, noninvasive, and easy-to-use bedside test (65). However, it relies on the assumption that subjects have similar body geometry as well as a constant composition of fat-free mass. Hydration status and changes relating to altered body configuration such as obesity may therefore significantly impact results (65,66). For estimating fat-free mass, single- and multifrequency impedance can be used and population-specific empirical regression models can be developed (65). BIA is considered a reasonably reliable screening test for body composition in healthy people with a body mass index (BMI) <34, while caution is advocated if BMI is higher (67). For dogs and cats, studies are few and the results are equivocal. In 22 cats, single-frequency BIA combined with defined zoometric measures was found to reliably predict fat-free mass by comparison with chemical analysis (68). Multifrequency BIA estimation of total body and extra-cellular water were compared with deuterium and bromide dilution estimations in cats in two studies (69,70). Both studies showed that the method was useful, but results depended on configuration ($r^2 = 0.17-0.71$) (69,70). In dogs, two studies have evaluated single-frequency BIA estimated body fat percentage compared with DEXA estimates (45,71). Despite a relatively good precision and correlation ($r^2 = 0.44-0.98$), imprecision varied between individual dogs and the agreement between methods were poor, resulting in the conclusion that agreement was unacceptable for clinical use without further validation (45,71).

4.5 ESTIMATING BODY COMPOSITION IN A CLINICAL SETTING

For initiating and monitoring weight-loss interventions in veterinary clinics, reliable methods to evaluate the patient's degree of obesity are necessary. In a practice setting it is seldom feasible to perform D_2O dilution, MRI, DEXA, or CT scans to assess body composition. It is time-consuming and expensive, and anesthesia or sedation is often not acceptable. Ideally, simple methods developed to estimate body composition should be accurate and precise, and it is important they should be fast and practical to perform in a first-opinion practice.

4.5.1 Body weight

Body weight (BW) can be objectively measured using a scale appropriate for the size of the animal. Ideally, the same scale should be used at each visit, as interscale variation may impact measurements. BW is easy to measure, gives an objective repeatable numerical result, and is an excellent tool for detecting subtle weight changes in the individual patient as well as for evaluating ongoing weight management programs. Therefore, BW should be recorded for all veterinary patients at all visits.

However, although BW accurately measures the total weight of the animal, its use for assessing body composition is limited (68,72,73). Ideal BW depends on breed, sex, exercise level, and stature, and differs between individuals, even within the same breed.

4.5.2 Morphometric measurements

4.5.2.1 BODY MASS INDEX (BMI)

Inspired by the human body mass index where an estimation of body composition is made based on an individual's height and weight, the feline and canine body mass indexes have been developed. Anthropometric measurements that provide a numerical evaluation of the body composition instead of the more rigid categorical results from body condition scoring evaluation is appealing, especially in research when more advanced methods are not available.

4.5.2.1.1 Canine BMI

For assessing the canine BMI and gender-specific body fat percentage (BF%), equations based on morphometric measurements have been proposed (74). According to the authors, the morphometric measurements were easy to perform with the dog standing squarely and looking straight ahead (46). BF% calculations showed a good correlation ($r^2 = 0.9-0.92$) and agreement with DEXA results, whereas BMI calculations, despite a significant correlation with DEXA ($r^2 = 0.54$), showed poor agreement for individual values (46,71). In a study performed on different genetic breeds of dogs, the correlation between BF% equations and DEXA results were lower ($r^2 = 0.49-0.58$), and agreement for individual measurements was unacceptable (71). Breed-specific calculations were for certain breeds better, and combining morphometric measures with BIA showed some promise, but more studies are needed on different genetic dog breeds to determine if global or breed-specific equations can reliably estimate body fat percentage in dogs.

4.5.2.1.2 Feline BMI

A feline body mass index (FBMI) has also been proposed (75,76). Hawthorne and Butterwick report that this method was a stronger predictor of BF% measured by DEXA ($r^2 = 0.85$) than body condition scoring ($r^2 = 0.73$) (76). In a recent study, we found a good correlation between BF% estimated by FBMI and by DEXA ($r^2 = 0.85$) (77), however, the two methods disagreed more than 10% for individual BF%, and measurements could easily vary a few centimeters depending on the cooperation from the cat. According to the FBMI instructions, the cat should be in a standing position, with legs perpendicular to the table and the head in an upright position (75). This pose is, in our experience, difficult to achieve, making the FBMI less useful in practice settings.

4.5.2.2 NOVEL MORPHOMETRIC EQUATIONS

New morphometric equations have been proposed by the University of Tennessee in collaboration with Hill's Pet Nutrition (Topeka, Kansas) (51,52). For dogs, the best-fit equations had adjusted r^2 of 0.98 for estimation of lean body mass (rather lean soft tissue mass as previously described in DEXA discussion and Figure 4.1), 0.98 for estimation of fat mass, and 0.82 for BF%. For cats, adjusted r^2 values were 0.85 for estimation of lean body mass and 0.98 for estimation of fat mass (52). The investigators found a relatively low interrater (1%–19.5%) and intrarater (<2%) variability for both systems and estimated that all measurements could be achieved within 5 minutes for the individual animal. However, some dogs and cats needed to be sedated to allow all measurements (51,52). Only a few cat breeds were included and also the wide range of size and conformation of domestic dogs in general presents a major challenge for developing standardized equations for assessing body composition. Thus, these morphometric equations remain to be validated in separate study populations to determine whether they are globally applicable in the pet populations.

4.5.3 Morphologic estimates

4.5.3.1 BODY CONDITION SCORING

Body condition scoring systems for dogs and cats are subjective semiquantitative methods that use visual and palpable characteristics to estimate the degree of obesity. Based on inspection and palpation of predefined fat depots, a BCS can be deduced from a defined scale. The fat covering of the ribcage, presence or absence of a waist, and size of the abdominal fat pad are often evaluated for assigning BCS in cats and dogs. Several scoring systems have been proposed (47,48,78–81). When using half points, the 5-point system is similar to the 9-point system (11). None of the proposed systems have been extensively validated, but the 5- and 9-point systems where 1 is emaciated, 3 or 5 is ideal, and 5 or 9 is grossly obese seem to be more extensively used (1,45,51,52,71–73,82–88). A BCS assigned according to the 9-point scale has shown good correlation with BF% measured by DEXA in both colony and client-owned cats ($r^2 = 0.64$–0.83) as well as colony and client-owned dogs ($r^2 = 0.58$–0.92) (45–49,73,78). Based on the initial development of the systems in cats and dogs, it was determined that dogs with an ideal BCS of 5/9 had $19 \pm 8\%$ fat mass, whereas in male cats a BCS of 5/9 related to $21.8 \pm 1.7\%$ fat mass, and that a 5% increase in fat mass was observed with each increase in BCS for both species (47,78,89). Despite similar correlations, however, the BF% relating to each BCS unit may differ between populations. In dogs, Mawby et al. found the ideal BCS of 5/9 to relate to $11 \pm 2\%$ fat mass and that each unit increase in BCS was associated with an 8.7% increase in fat mass (46). A study from our group found that indoor-confined, neutered client-owned male and female cats with a BCS 5/9 had a median of 31.8% BF (range 23.6%–38.4% BF) and each unit increment was 5%–6% (49), whereas in another study a BCS of 3/5 equated with $11.7 \pm 4.5\%$ BF and a ½ unit BCS increase equaled 7% BF in a colony cat facility (73). The use of different DEXA hardware and software systems or differences in body condition scoring technique by individual researchers could be part of the reason for the reported differences in BF% levels. In previous studies, however, both intraobserver CV (8.1%) and interobserver CV (11.6%–15%) were relatively low for body condition scoring (47,48). Differences between studies could relate to indoor-confined sedentary pets being sarcopenic (having decreased muscle mass) compared with colony populations or pets with outdoor access (90) and differences in selection of populations included in individual studies is likely to impact results. For dogs, the large variation in breed standards affect the correlation between BCS and BF%. For an ideal BCS of 5/9, greyhounds had significantly less body fat (7.2%) than huskies (31%) and tended to have less fat than rottweilers (32%), while the difference was not significant compared with poodles (18%) and dachshunds (15%) (71). Further, depending on breed, each unit increase in BCS was associated with an average increase of 1.5% BF–6.5% BF. These findings highlight the importance of developing breed-specific BCS charts. Size-specific charts including illustrations of all nine body condition scores have been proposed by Royal Canin (91), but these have to the authors knowledge not yet been validated.

It should be noted that all BCS systems have been developed and validated on populations including no or very few animals with a BCS <4/9 and relatively low numbers with BCS above 8/9, and studies have only included animals with a fat mass of up to 45% for BCS 9/9 or 5/5 (46,47,49,71,73,78,89).

Recently, the 5-point BCS system was evaluated in relation to the development of a canine and feline body fat index (BFI) where it was found to be inferior to the proposed systems (51,52). By definition, all animals assigned a BCS 5/5 were assessed to have 40% BF with the BCS system used. The poor performance of the BCS in this study, therefore, more likely reflects the fact that 65% of the dogs and 71% of the cats in the selected populations had a BF% >40%, for all of which BF% would naturally be underestimated according to the definitions used.

The accuracy of body condition scoring relies significantly on investigator training. Veterinarians or trained scorers provide a more accurate BCS compared with untrained scorers or owners, where the latter often underestimate their pet's BCS (2,4,5,73). In one study, implementing a 5-point BCS system for owner evaluation of their pet's body condition did not improve agreement with a trained investigator (3). Further studies are needed for evaluating how to best educate owners in identifying and monitoring weight changes in their pets.

The BCS systems are easy to use in a clinical setting; are illustrative and repeatable; and provide valuable tools for assessing if a pet is normal weight, underweight, or overweight. Further, they complement body weight measures in planning and monitoring individual weight loss programs (92). However, cats and dogs with a BCS of 9 may display a wide range of body fat percentages, making it challenging to accurately determine ideal body weight for these patients.

4.5.3.2 CANINE AND FELINE BODY FAT INDEX (BFI)

To address the problem of assessing BF% in grossly obese pets, two supplemental systems have been developed and validated for cats and dogs respectively (51,52). These systems are also based on inspection and palpation at predefined areas of the animal's body. They cover animals from mildly overweight (BFI 30; BF% 25–35) to extremely obese (BFI 60; BF% 56–65). The cat or dog can be categorized according to six illustrations and written descriptions, and the ideal BW is then estimated from a chart based on the current weight and BFI category (51,52). The investigators found that BF% estimated with the BFI system was within 10% of the value determined via DEXA for 53% of the dogs and within 20% of the DEXA value for 91% of the dogs. Body fat percentage predicted with the BFI was within 10% of the DEXA value for 56% of the cats and within 20% of the DEXA value for 90% of the cats. Correlation between methods was not reported. Only few of the included dogs and cats were underweight or lean (5 dogs [6%] with BF% <25 and 6 cats [8%] with BF% <30), and the intended application of both BFI systems is therefore as a complement to BCS when an overweight or obese dog or cat is identified.

4.6 CLINICAL RECOMMENDATIONS FOR GENERAL PRACTICE

Body condition scoring systems complement bodyweight monitoring in identifying pets at risk of developing obesity at a stage where prevention measures can be more easily implemented. In veterinary practices it should be emphasized to implement weighing and assessment of body composition in all consultations with actions taken on deviations from ideal. Especially following neutering, owners should be advised on decreasing food allowance as well as monitoring their pet's weight regularly. Muscle condition scoring systems have been proposed and ideally complement the BCS systems, however, their use in obesity treatment need to be further developed and validated (10,50).

Possibly BIA, eventually in combination with morphometric measurements, could provide more accurate and precise methods to estimate fat-free mass in both cats and dogs of different breeds and housing, but this remains to be further studied. In humans, BMI is used to estimate the health risk linked to obesity in an individual. In cats and dogs there are currently no defined degrees of obesity that link to risk of disease, but in Labrador retrievers a fat mass above 25% has been associated with increased insulin resistance, osteoarthritis, and a shorter lifespan (58,93,94), while obesity in cats is known to predispose to insulin resistance and diabetes mellitus (95,96) (see Chapter 3).

4.7 CONCLUSION

To prevent and treat obesity in pets, easy and reliable systems for assessment of body composition are pivotal. If advanced methods such as D_2O, DEXA, CT, or MRI are unavailable, the 5- or 9-point body condition scoring systems have repeatedly shown acceptable performances in identifying obesity in dogs and cats. However, overlapping scores and discrepancies between BCS and mean body fat percentage limits the systems' applicability in obesity research. Further, the newly developed BFI should probably be preferred for estimating optimal BW in grossly obese subjects.

REFERENCES

1. Courcier EA, O'Higgins R, Mellor DJ, Yam PS. Prevalence and risk factors for feline obesity in a first opinion practice in Glasgow, Scotland. *Journal of Feline Medicine and Surgery* 2010;12(10):746–53.
2. Courcier EA, Mellor DJ, Thomson RM, Yam PS. A cross sectional study of the prevalence and risk factors for owner misperception of canine body shape in first opinion practice in Glasgow. *Preventive Veterinary Medicine* 2011;102(1):66–74.
3. Eastland-Jones RC, German AJ, Holden SL, Biourge V, Pickavance LC. Owner misperception of canine body condition persists despite use of a body condition score chart. *Journal of Nutritional Science* 2014;3:e45.

4. Colliard L, Ancel J, Benet JJ, Paragon BM, Blanchard G. Risk factors for obesity in dogs in France. *Journal of Nutrition* 2006;136(7 Suppl): 1951S–1954S.

5. Colliard L, Paragon BM, Lemuet B, Benet JJ, Blanchard G. Prevalence and risk factors of obesity in an urban population of healthy cats. *Journal of Feline Medicine and Surgery* 2009;11(2):135–40.

6. Remillard RL, Darden DE, Michel KE, Marks SL, Buffington CA, Bunnell PR. An investigation of the relationship between caloric intake and outcome in hospitalized dogs. *Veterinary Therapeutics: Research in Applied Veterinary Medicine* 2001;2(4):301–10.

7. Burkholder WJ. Use of body condition scores in clinical assessment of the provision of optimal nutrition. *Journal of the American Veterinary Medical Association* 2000;217(5):650–4.

8. Lund EM, Armstrong P, Kirk CA, Klausner J. Prevalence and risk factors for obesity in adult cats from private US veterinary practices. *International Journal of Applied Research in Veterinary Medicine* 2005;3(2):88–96.

9. Bjornvad CR, Kristensen AT, Jessen LR, Annerud K. Nutritional management of veterinary hospitalized patients in Denmark. *Research Abstract Program of the 25th Annual ACVIM Forum*. Seattle, WA. 2007.

10. Freeman L, Becvarova I, Cave N et al. WSAVA global nutrition assessment guidelines. *Journal of Small Animal Practice* 2011;00(June):1–12.

11. Brooks D, Churchill J, Fein K et al. 2014 AAHA weight management guidelines for dogs and cats. *Journal of the American Animal Hospital Association* 2014;50(1):1–11.

12. Speakman JR, Booles D, Butterwick R. Validation of dual energy x-ray absorptiometry (DXA) by comparison with chemical analysis of dogs and cats. *International Journal of Obesity* 2001;25(3):439–47.

13. Burkholder WJ, Thatcher CD. Validation of predictive equations for use of deuterium oxide dilution to determine body composition of dogs. *American Journal of Veterinary Research* 1998;59(8):927–37.

14. Munday HS. Assessment of body composition in cats and dogs. *International Journal of Obesity* 1994;18:S14–S21.

15. Jensen MD. Research techniques for body composition assessment. *Journal of the American Dietetic Association* 1992;92(4):454–60.

16. Jebb SA. Measurement of soft tissue composition by dual energy x-ray absorptiometry. *The British Journal of Nutrition* 1997;77(2):151–63.

17. Plank LD. Dual-energy x-ray absorptiometry and body composition. *Current Opinion in Clinical Nutrition and Metabolic Care* 2005;8(3):305–309.

18. Grier SJ, Turner AS, Alvis MR. The use of dual-energy x-ray absorptiometry in animals. *Investigative Radiology* 1996;31(1):50–62.

19. Wang ZM, Pierson RN, Jr., Heymsfield SB. The five-level model: A new approach to organizing body-composition research. *American Journal of Clinical Nutrition* 1992;56(1):19–28.

20. Pietrobelli A, Formica C, Wang Z, Heymsfield SB. Dual-energy x-ray absorptiometry body composition model: Review of physical concepts. *American Journal of Physiology* 1996;271(6 Pt 1):E941–51.
21. Heymsfield SB, Wang Z, Baumgartner RN, Ross R. Human body composition: Advances in models and methods. *Annual Review of Nutrition* 1997;17:527–58.
22. Genton L, Hans D, Kyle UG, Pichard C. Dual-energy x-ray absorptiometry and body composition: Differences between devices and comparison with reference methods. *Nutrition* 2002;18(1):66–70.
23. Tothill P, Avenell A, Reid DM. Precision and accuracy of measurements of whole-body bone mineral: Comparisons between Hologic, Lunar and Norland dual-energy x-ray absorptiometers. *The British Journal of Radiology* 1994;67(804):1210–7.
24. Tothill P, Avenell A, Love J, Reid DM. Comparisons between Hologic, Lunar and Norland dual-energy x-ray absorptiometers and other techniques used for whole-body soft tissue measurements. *European Journal of Clinical Nutrition* 1994;48(11):781–94.
25. Sakai Y, Ito H, Meno T, Numata M, Jingu S. Comparison of body composition measurements obtained by two fan-beam DXA instruments. *Journal of Clinical Densitometry* 2006;9(2):191–7.
26. Lauten SD, Cox NR, Brawner WR, Baker HJ. Use of dual energy x-ray absorptiometry for noninvasive body composition measurements in clinically normal dogs. *American Journal of Veterinary Research* 2001;62(8):1295–301.
27. Svendsen OL, Haarbo J, Hassager C, Christiansen C. Accuracy of measurements of body composition by dual-energy x-ray absorptiometry in vivo. *The American Journal of Clinical Nutrition* 1993;57(5):605–8.
28. Brunton JA, Bayley HS, Atkinson SA. Validation and application of dual-energy x-ray absorptiometry to measure bone mass and body composition in small infants. *The American Journal of Clinical Nutrition* 1993;58(6):839–45.
29. Pintauro SJ, Nagy TR, Duthie CM, Goran MI. Cross-calibration of fat and lean measurements by dual-energy x-ray absorptiometry to pig carcass analysis in the pediatric body weight range. *American Journal of Clinical Nutrition* 1996;63(3):293–8.
30. Mitchell AD, Conway JM, Potts WJE. Body composition analysis of pigs by dual-energy x-ray absorptiometry. *Journal of Animal Science* 1996;74(11):2663–71.
31. Picaud JC, Rigo J, Nyamugabo K, Milet J, Senterre J. Evaluation of dual-energy x-ray absorptiometry for body-composition assessment in piglets and term human neonates. *American Journal of Clinical Nutrition* 1996;63(2):157–63.
32. Ellis KJ, Shypailo RJ, Pratt JA, Pond WG. Accuracy of dual-energy x-ray absorptiometry for body-composition measurements in children. *The American Journal of Clinical Nutrition* 1994;60(5):660–5.

33. Mitchell AD, Scholz AM, Conway JM. Body composition analysis of small pigs by dual-energy x-ray absorptiometry. *Journal of Animal Science* 1998;76(9):2392–8.

34. Black A, Tilmont EM, Baer DJ, Rumpler DK, Roth GS, Lane MA. Accuracy and precision of dual-energy x-ray absorptiometry for body composition measurements in rhesus monkeys. *Journal of Medical Primatology* 2001;30(2):94–99.

35. Son HR, d'Avignon A, Laflamme DP. Comparison of dual-energy x-ray absorptiometry and measurement of total body water content by deuterium oxide dilution for estimating body composition in dogs. *American Journal of Veterinary Research* 1998;59(5):529–32.

36. Koo WW, Hammami M, Hockman EM. Use of fan beam dual energy x-ray absorptiometry to measure body composition of piglets. *The Journal of Nutrition* 2002;132(6):1380–3.

37. Brunton JA, Weiler HA, Atkinson SA. Improvement in the accuracy of dual energy x-ray absorptiometry for whole body and regional analysis of body composition: Validation using piglets and methodologic considerations in infants. *Pediatric Research* 1997;41(4):590–6.

38. Munday HS, Booles D, Anderson P, Poore DW, Earle KE. The repeatability of body composition measurements in dogs and cats using dual energy x-ray absorptiometry. *The Journal of Nutrition* 1994;124(12 Suppl):2619s–21s.

39. Toll PW, Gross KL, Berryhill SA, Jewell DE. Usefulness of dual energy x-ray absorptiometry for body composition measurement in adult dogs. *The Journal of Nutrition* 1994;124(12 Suppl):2601S–2603S.

40. Lauten SD, Cox NR, Baker GH, Painter DJ, Morrison NE, Baker HJ. Body composition of growing and adult cats as measured by use of dual energy x-ray absorptiometry. *Comparative Medicine* 2000;50(2):175–83.

41. German AJ, Holden S, Bissot T, Morris PJ, Biourge V. Changes in body composition during weight loss in obese client-owned cats: Loss of lean tissue mass correlates with overall percentage of weight lost. *Journal of Feline Medicine and Surgery* 2008;10(5):452–9.

42. Munday HS, Earle KE, Anderson P. Changes in the body composition of the domestic shorthaired cat during growth and development. *The Journal of Nutrition* 1994;124(12 Suppl):2622S–2623S.

43. Mosing M, German AJ, Holden SL et al. Oxygenation and ventilation characteristics in obese sedated dogs before and after weight loss: A clinical trial. *Veterinary Journal* 2013;198(2):367–71.

44. Vitger AD, Stallknecht BM, Nielsen DH, Bjornvad CR. Integration of a physical training program in a weight loss plan for overweight pet dogs. *Journal of the American Veterinary Medical Association* 2016;248(2):174–82.

45. German AJ, Holden SL, Morris PJ, Biourge V. Comparison of a bioimpedance monitor with dual-energy x-ray absorptiometry for noninvasive estimation of percentage body fat in dogs. *American Journal of Veterinary Research* 2010;71(4):393–8.

46. Mawby DI, Bartges JW, d'Avignon A, Laflamme DP, Moyers TD, Cottrell T. Comparison of various methods for estimating body fat in dogs. *Journal of the American Animal Hospital Association* 2004;40(2):109–14.

47. Laflamme D. Development and validation of a body condition score system for cats: A clinical tool. *Feline Practice* 1997;25(5/6):13–18.

48. German AJ, Holden SL, Moxham GL, Holmes KL, Hackett RM, Rawlings JM. A simple, reliable tool for owners to assess the body condition of their dog or cat. *The Journal of Nutrition* 2006;136(7):2031S–2033S.

49. Bjornvad CR, Nielsen DH, Armstrong PJ et al. Evaluation of a nine-point body condition scoring system in physically inactive pet cats. *American Journal of Veterinary Research* 2011;72(4):433–7.

50. Michel KE, Anderson W, Cupp C, Laflamme DP. Correlation of a feline muscle mass score with body composition determined by dual-energy x-ray absorptiometry. *British Journal of Nutrition* 2011;106(Suppl 1): S57–S59.

51. Witzel AL, Kirk CA, Henry GA, Toll PW, Brejda JJ, Paetau-Robinson I. Use of a novel morphometric method and body fat index system for estimation of body composition in overweight and obese dogs. *Journal of the American Veterinary Medical Association* 2014;244(11):1279–84.

52. Witzel AL, Kirk CA, Henry GA, Toll PW, Brejda JJ, Paetau-Robinson I. Use of a morphometric method and body fat index system for estimation of body composition in overweight and obese cats. *Journal of the American Veterinary Medical Association* 2014;244(11):1285–90.

53. Bushberg JT. *The Essential Physics of Medical Imaging*. 3rd ed. Philadelphia: Lippincott Williams & Wilkins; 2011.

54. Ishioka K, Okumura M, Sagawa M, Nakadomo F, Kimura K, Saito M. Computed tomographic assessment of body fat in beagles. *Veterinary Radiology & Ultrasound* 2005;46(1):49–53.

55. Lee H, Kim M, Choi M et al. Assessment of feline abdominal adipose tissue using computed tomography. *Journal of Feline Medicine and Surgery* 2010;12(12):936–41.

56. Buelund LE, Nielsen DH, McEvoy FJ, Svalastoga EL, Bjornvad CR. Measurement of body composition in cats using computed tomography and dual energy x-ray absorptiometry. *Veterinary Radiology & Ultrasound* 2011;52(2):179–84.

57. Kobayashi T, Koie H, Kusumi A, Kitagawa M, Kanayama K, Otsuji K. Comparative investigation of body composition in male dogs using CT and body fat analysis software. *The Journal of Veterinary Medical Science* 2014;76(3):439–46.

58. Muller L, Kollar E, Balogh L et al. Body fat distribution and metabolic consequences: Examination opportunities in dogs. *Acta Veterinaria Hungarica* 2014;62(2):169–79.

59. Hoenig M, Thomaseth K, Waldron M, Ferguson DC. Insulin sensitivity, fat distribution, and adipocytokine response to different diets in lean and obese cats before and after weight loss. *American Journal of Physiology: Regulatory, Integrative and Comparative Physiology* 2007;292(1):R227–34.

60. Gifford A, Kullberg J, Berglund J et al. Canine body composition quantification using 3 tesla fat-water MRI. *Journal of Magnetic Resonance Imaging* 2014;39(2):485–91.

61. Zanghi BM, Cupp CJ, Pan YL et al. Noninvasive measurements of body composition and body water via quantitative magnetic resonance, deuterium water, and dual-energy x-ray absorptiometry in awake and sedated dogs. *American Journal of Veterinary Research* 2013;74(5):733–43.

62. Zanghi BM, Cupp CJ, Pan YL et al. Noninvasive measurements of body composition and body water via quantitative magnetic resonance, deuterium water, and dual-energy x-ray absorptiometry in cats. *American Journal of Veterinary Research* 2013;74(5):721–32.

63. Ballevre O, Anantharaman-Barr G, Gicquello P, Piguet-Welsh C, Thielin AL, Fern E. Use of the doubly-labeled water method to assess energy expenditure in free living cats and dogs. *Journal of Nutrition* 1994;124(12 Suppl):2594S–2600S.

64. Speakman JR, Perez-Camargo G, McCappin T, Frankel T, Thomson P, Legrand-Defretin V. Validation of the doubly-labelled water technique in the domestic dog (*Canis familiaris*). *British Journal of Nutrition* 2001;85(1):75–87.

65. Kyle UG, Bosaeus I, De Lorenzo AD et al. Bioelectrical impedance analysis—Part I: Review of principles and methods. *Clinical Nutrition* 2004;23(5):1226–43.

66. Lukaski HC. Evolution of bioimpedance: A circuitous journey from estimation of physiological function to assessment of body composition and a return to clinical research. *European Journal of Clinical Nutrition* 2013;67(Suppl 1):S2–S9.

67. Kyle UG, Bosaeus I, De Lorenzo AD et al. Bioelectrical impedance analysis-part II: utilization in clinical practice. *Clinical Nutrition* 2004;23(6):1430–53.

68. Stanton CA, Hamar DW, Johnson DE, Fettman MJ. Bioelectrical impedance and zoometry for body composition analysis in domestic cats. *American Journal of Veterinary Research* 1992;53(2):251–7.

69. Elliott DA, Backus RC, Van Loan MD, Rogers QR. Evaluation of multifrequency bioelectrical impedance analysis for the assessment of extracellular and total body water in healthy cats. *Journal of Nutrition* 2002;132(6 Suppl 2):1757S–1759S.

70. Elliott DA, Backus RC, Van Loan MD, Rogers QR. Extracellular water and total body water estimated by multifrequency bioelectrical impedance analysis in healthy cats: A cross-validation study. *Journal of Nutrition* 2002;132(6 Suppl 2):1760S–1762S.

71. Jeusette I, Greco D, Aquino F et al. Effect of breed on body composition and comparison between various methods to estimate body composition in dogs. *Research in Veterinary Science* 2010;88(2):227–32.

72. Kienzle E, Moik K. A pilot study of the body weight of pure-bred client-owned adult cats. *The British Journal of Nutrition* 2011;106(Suppl 1): S113–S115.

73. Shoveller AK, DiGennaro J, Lanman C, Spangler D. Trained vs untrained evaluator assessment of body condition score as a predictor of percent body fat in adult cats. *Journal of Feline Medicine and Surgery* 2014;16(12):957–65.

74. Burkholder W, Toll P. Obesity. In: Hand MS, Thatcher CD, Remillard RL, Roudebush P, editors. *Small Animal Clinical Nutrition*. 4th ed. Topeka, KS: Mark Morris Institute; 2000, pp. 401–430.

75. Butterwick R. How fat is that cat? *Journal of Feline Medicine and Surgery* 2000;2(2):91–94.

76. Hawthorne A, Butterwick R. Predicting the body composition of cats: Development of a zoometric measurement for estimation of percentage body fat in cats [abstract]. *Journal of Veterinary Internal Medicine* 2000;14(3):365.

77. Falkenberg M, Hoelmkjaer KM, Cronin A, Nielsen DH, Bjornvad CR. Evaluering af overensstemmelsen af body condition score og feline body mass index sammenlignet med dual energy x-ray absorptiometry hos katte. *Dansk Veterinaertidsskrift* 2016;4:32–37.

78. Laflamme D. Development and validation of a body condition score system for dogs. *Canine Practice* 1997;22(4):10–15.

79. Edney AT, Smith PM. Study of obesity in dogs visiting veterinary practices in the United Kingdom. *Veterinary Record* 1986;118(14):391–6.

80. Diez M. Body condition scoring in cats and dogs. *Waltham Focus* 2006;16(1):39–40.

81. Scarlett JM, Donoghue S, Saidla J, Wills J. Overweight cats: Prevalence and risk factors. *International Journal of Obesity and Related Metabolic Disorders* 1994;18(Suppl 1):S22–S28.

82. Corbee RJ. Obesity in show cats. *Journal of Animal Physiology and Animal Nutrition* 2014;98(6):1075–80.

83. Corbee RJ. Obesity in show dogs. *Journal of Animal Physiology and Animal Nutrition* 2013;97(5):904–10.

84. Scott KC, Levy JK, Gorman SP, Newell SM. Body condition of feral cats and the effect of neutering. *Journal of Applied Animal Welfare Science* 2002;5(3):203–13.

85. Weeth LP, Fascetti AJ, Kass PH, Suter SE, Santos AM, Delaney SJ. Prevalence of obese dogs in a population of dogs with cancer. *American Journal of Veterinary Research* 2007;68(4):389–98.

86. Yaissle JE, Holloway C, Buffington CA. Evaluation of owner education as a component of obesity treatment programs for dogs. *Journal of the American Veterinary Medical Association* 2004;224(12):1932–5.

87. Kronfeld DS, Donoghue S, Glickman LT. Body condition of cats. *Journal of Nutrition* 1994;124(12 Suppl):2683S–2684S.

88. Baez JL, Michel KE, Sorenmo K, Shofer FS. A prospective investigation of the prevalence and prognostic significance of weight loss and changes in body condition in feline cancer patients. *Journal of Feline Medicine and Surgery* 2007;9(5):411–7.
89. Laflamme D. Estimation of body fat by body condition score. *Journal of Veterinary Internal Medicine* 1994;8(2):154.
90. Cline MG, Witzel AL, Moyers TD, Bartges JW, Kirk CA. Body composition of outdoor-intact cats compared to indoor-neutered cats using dual energy x-ray absorptiometry [abstract]. *Journal of Animal Physiology and Animal Nutrition* 2013;97(6):1191.
91. Royal Canin. Body condition charts [December 11, 2015]. Available from: http://www.royalcaninhealthyweight.co.uk/pet-obesity.
92. German AJ, Holden SL, Bissot T, Morris PJ, Biourge V. Use of starting condition score to estimate changes in body weight and composition during weight loss in obese dogs. *Research in Veterinary Science* 2009;87(2):249–54.
93. Lawler DF, Larson BT, Ballam JM et al. Diet restriction and ageing in the dog: Major observations over two decades. *British Journal of Nutrition* 2008;99(4):793–805.
94. Smith GK, Paster ER, Powers MY et al. Lifelong diet restriction and radiographic evidence of osteoarthritis of the hip joint in dogs. *Journal of the American Veterinary Medical Association* 2006;229(5):690–3.
95. Sallander M, Eliasson J, Hedhammar A. Prevalence and risk factors for the development of diabetes mellitus in Swedish cats. *Acta Veterinaria Scandinavica* 2012;54:61.
96. Bjornvad CR, Rand JS, Tan HY et al. Obesity and sex influence insulin resistance and total and multimer adiponectin levels in adult neutered domestic shorthair client-owned cats. *Domestic Animal Endocrinology* 2014;47:55–64.

5

Nutritional management of obesity

MARTHA G. CLINE AND MARYANNE MURPHY

Patients with excess body weight require dedicated time to address diet history, and nutritional and exercise recommendations in addition to the patient evaluation. This process starts with an accurate diagnosis of obesity and subsequent estimation of target body weight (TBW) or ideal body weight (IBW). Current caloric intake and estimated energy requirements for weight loss are compared prior to making a diet selection and weight loss program recommendations. Consistent reevaluation, including after TBW has been achieved, gives cats and dogs the best chance at long-term success.

5.1 PATIENT EVALUATION

5.1.1 Diagnosis of obesity

When obesity occurs, the veterinary team is tasked with ruling out and appropriately addressing any comorbidities (see Chapter 3) and accurately diagnosing the condition via body composition evaluation (see Chapter 4). When weight and body condition score (BCS) (Figure 5.1) indicate overweight or obesity, both the pet owner and veterinary team must recognize and discuss possible treatment options for this medical condition. Surveys of dogs and cats presenting to veterinarians in primary or referral practices indicate that only 11.4% of overweight/obese dogs and 3.6% of overweight/obese cats have overweight or obesity listed as a medical problem (1,2). Further, many pet owners underestimate their pet's BCS and those who recognize a high BCS tend not to consider these pets to be overweight (3–5) (see Chapter 6).

Every increase in the 9-point BCS scale is equivalent to an approximately 5% increase in body fat (BF) (6,7) (Table 5.1). Cats and dogs can be considered overweight with a BCS of 6–7/9 (approximately 25%–34% BF) and obese ≥8/9 (approximately ≥35% BF). The BCS system includes animals up to 45% BF, but measurements have been reported to be as high as 62% BF in cats and 65% BF in dogs (8,9). Each BCS on the 9-point scale can also be associated with an approximately 10% increase in excess body weight (Table 5.1) (6,7,10). Since animals can be >40% overweight or >45% BF, additional tools may help both pet owners and the veterinary team more accurately diagnose obesity. The body fat index (BFI) (Figure 5.2) has been designed to determine an estimated body fat percentage (BF%) via use of written descriptors, selected based on palpation, for animals up to 65% BF (8,9) (see Chapter 4). Using these tools in the exam room and inviting the owner to participate in the palpation of their animal is a useful way to help the owner recognize their pet's overweight or obese status and reaffirm the diagnosis of this medical condition.

5.1.2 Estimating target or ideal body weight

An essential part of weight management is establishing a TBW or IBW for the patient. The TBW represents the weight the veterinary team is aiming to achieve as part of the weight loss program. This value may differ from the IBW if a loss to IBW is considered inappropriate. This is usually the result of a comorbidity to obesity such as cardiovascular or kidney disease. Ideal body weight can be determined from historic data when medical records include both body weight and BCS. Equations are also available to estimate ideal body weight using BF%, percentage of excess body weight, or BCS (Box 5.1) (11,12). Clinically practical ways to estimate BF% include BCS, BFI, or morphometric measurements (6–9,13). Predictive equations using morphometric measurements can be used to predict body fat mass, lean body mass, and BF% (Box 5.2) (8,9). The authors typically reserve the use of morphometric measurements for cats and dogs with obesity and a good disposition.

It is important to note that BCS and BFI account for body fat and not lean body mass. As animals age, they may develop sarcopenia, the loss of muscle mass that occurs with age unrelated to an underlying inflammatory or pathologic condition (14). In older dogs, sarcopenia may be most evident along the epaxial musculature as opposed to temporal and quadriceps muscle measurements (15). Muscle condition score (MCS) is recommended as part of a complete nutritional assessment by the World Small Animal Veterinary Association (WSAVA) and includes palpation and visualization of the temporal bones, scapula, ribs, lumbar vertebrae, and pelvic bones (Figure 5.3) (16). Although this system is not validated to lean body mass, especially in relation to obesity, it can be used to subjectively assess muscle loss with good repeatability, particularly when performed by the same assessor over time (17). Because the percentage of lean body mass impacts BF%, in animals with a degree of age-related muscle atrophy, an ideal BF% of 25 may be acceptable.

5.2 ENERGY REQUIREMENTS FOR WEIGHT MANAGEMENT

5.2.1 Determining current caloric intake

To successfully manage an overweight or obese patient, an estimation of the patient's current caloric intake must be determined. Clinicians should specifically question pet owners about a variety of foods to ensure all sources of caloric intake are accounted for (Box 5.3). A comprehensive diet, activity, and household history form (DAHHF; see Chapter 8, Appendix 8.1) can be completed by the pet owner and used by the veterinary staff to calculate current intake levels. Owners can complete the DAHHF either before an appointment to discuss weight loss or after an appointment where overweight or obesity is identified, due to the time needed to properly complete the form.

Caloric content of commercial products can be found by referencing the label, calling the manufacturer, or utilizing online resources. Under the Model Bill and Regulations PF9 in the Association of American Feed Control Officials (AAFCO) Official Publication, labels of dog or cat food, including, snacks, treats, and supplements, are required to have a statement of calorie content (18). Some chews and bones, including hooves, ears, pizzle sticks, and ligaments, are exempt from AAFCO label requirements unless the manufacturer makes a claim of nutrition value on the label. The Fédération européenne de l'industrie des aliments pour animaux familiers (FEDIAF) does not currently impose an energy content labeling requirement for European pet foods. The caloric content of most human food products can be found in the United States Department of Agriculture (USDA) nutrient database (19). Once total caloric intake is determined, it is compared to the patient's estimated energy requirements.

To ensure estimates of current caloric intake are as accurate as possible and to offer the best feeding advice moving forward, veterinary staff should obtain specific information about food bowls and measuring devices used by the owner. Sometimes obtaining an accurate diet history is difficult, if not impossible. Fortunately, most feeding practices by dog owners prior to weight loss do not

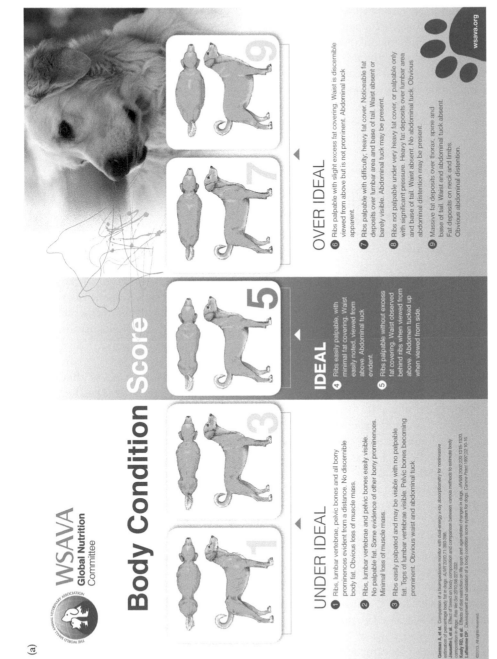

Figure 5.1 **(a, b)** Canine and feline body condition scoring system (9-point scale). (Global Nutrition Committee Toolkit courtesy of the World Small Animal Veterinary Association.)

(Continued)

(b)

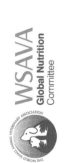

WSAVA
Global Nutrition Committee

wsava.org

Body Condition Score

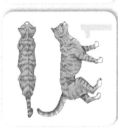

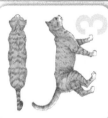

UNDER IDEAL

1. Ribs visible on shorthaired cats. No palpable fat. Severe abdominal tuck. Lumbar vertebrae and wings of ilia easily palpated.

2. Ribs easily visible on shorthaired cats. Lumbar vertebrae obvious. Pronounced abdominal tuck. No palpable fat.

3. Ribs easily palpable with minimal fat covering. Lumbar vertebrae obvious. Obvious waist behind ribs. Minimal abdominal fat

IDEAL

4. Ribs palpable with minimal fat covering. Noticeable waist behind ribs. Slight abdominal tuck. Abdominal fat pad absent.

5. Well-proportioned. Observe waist behind ribs. Ribs palpable with slight fat covering. Abdominal fat pad minimal.

OVER IDEAL

6. Ribs palpable with slight excess fat covering. Waist and abdominal fat pad distinguishable but not obvious. Abdominal tuck absent.

7. Ribs not easily palpated with moderate fat covering. Waist poorly discernible. Obvious rounding of abdomen. Moderate abdominal fat pad.

8. Ribs not palpable with excess fat covering. Waist absent. Obvious rounding of abdomen with prominent abdominal fat pad. Fat deposits present over lumbar area.

9. Ribs not palpable under heavy fat cover. Heavy fat deposits over lumbar area, face and limbs. Distention of abdomen with no waist. Extensive abdominal fat deposits.

Bjornvad CR, et al. Evaluation of a nine-point body condition scoring system in physically inactive pet cats. AJVR 2011;72:433-437 **Laflamme DP.** Development and validation of a body condition score system for cats. A clinical tool. Feline Pract 1997;25:13-18

©2013. All rights reserved.

Figure 5.1 (*Continued*)

Table 5.1 Relationship between body condition score with body fat percentage and excess body weight

BCS (9-point scale)	Body fat %	% Excess body weight
4	15–19	
5	20–24	
6	25–29	10
7	30–34	20
8	35–39	30
9	40+	40

Source: Brooks D et al., *Journal of the American Animal Hospital Association* 2014;50:1–11.

influence the success of a weight management program (20). If the veterinary staff members are unable to obtain a complete diet history, the program can still be instituted based on estimated energy requirements for weight loss.

5.2.2 Determining caloric intake for weight loss

There are several methods to estimate initial caloric intake for weight loss (Box 5.4) (11,21–23). The linear equation is not advised to calculate resting energy requirements (RER) in patients with an IBW under 2 kg or over 25 kg, as it will overestimate their caloric requirement (Figure 5.4). Specific factors can be used to adjust the calculated RER or maintenance energy requirement (MER) based on IBW or TBW. The energy intake needed to achieve weight loss in dogs has been reported as $63 \pm 10.2 \, \text{kcal}/\text{TBW}_{kg}^{0.75}/\text{day}$ (22). In cats, $52 \pm 4.9 \, \text{kcal}/\text{TBW}_{kg}^{0.711}/\text{day}$ is needed (23).

If current caloric intake is less than the calculated caloric intake for weight loss, it is advisable to reduce current caloric intake by 10%–20%. The authors typically do not advise restricting below $42.6 \, \text{kcal}/\text{TBW}_{kg}^{0.75}/\text{day}$ in dogs or $42.2 \, \text{kcal}/\text{TBW}_{kg}^{0.711}/\text{day}$ in cats (approximately 60% RER) (22,23). If this type of caloric restriction is required, screening for underlying confounding comorbidities (see Chapter 3) or consulting with a Board Certified Veterinary Nutritionist™ is recommended to avoid potential complication from nutritional deficiencies. One study evaluated the theoretical risk of nutrient deficiency in three over-the-counter (OTC) and two therapeutic weight management diets for dogs when the diets were fed under caloric restriction (24). All diets had at least one essential nutrient deficiency at $79 \, \text{kcal}/\text{kg}^{0.75}/\text{day}$ and multiple deficiencies at $70 \, \text{kcal}/\text{kg}^{0.75}/\text{day}$. The therapeutic weight management diets had fewer nutrient deficiencies at each level of restriction when compared to the OTC diets, and the most common nutrient deficiencies were choline and selenium. In a follow-up study, decreased plasma choline was documented in dogs following a weight loss program while on a therapeutic weight loss diet. However, no signs of choline deficiency were documented, most nutrients did not change significantly, and the dogs remained apparently healthy throughout their weight loss program (25).

For animals with an accurate diet history and known caloric consumption, some practitioners may elect to decrease the animal's current caloric intake by 20% to avoid sudden and drastic reductions in caloric intake. In these cases, the rate of weight loss may be slow or unsuccessful if the pet was gaining weight prior to this reduction. While this method may be more conservative, challenges with owner adherence and frustration due to lack of success should be considered. Successful weight loss at subsequent visits is an excellent motivator for owner adherence, and subjective owner descriptions of food-seeking behavior have been shown to decrease in dogs on the more typical caloric restriction weight loss program (22). Cats, however, have been shown to both increase and decrease food-seeking behavior when consuming a restricted energy level (23,26,27).

Regardless of the method used to determine IBW/TBW and calculate energy requirements, these are initial estimates that may change over time. Follow-up is necessary to tailor the pet's weight loss program based on their individual metabolic requirements and to reassess their body condition to determine when TBW is achieved.

5.3 IMPLEMENTATION OF A TREATMENT PROGRAM

5.3.1 Diet selection

5.3.1.1 MACRONUTRIENTS

A therapeutic weight management diet is recommended for animals with obesity undergoing significant caloric restriction. These types of diets are high in protein to promote satiety and maintenance of lean body mass during weight loss, while avoiding protein deficiency with caloric restriction. Therapeutic weight management diets, particularly for dogs, also contain high levels of fiber and low caloric density for an additional satiety effect. These diets are fortified in micronutrients to avoid potential deficiencies that may occur with caloric restriction.

Protein is the most satiating macronutrient and is able to increase energy expenditure due to the energetic cost of protein synthesis and gluconeogenesis. Excess protein may also be provided in high enough levels to maintain adequate protein intake despite overall energy restriction (28,29). Beagle dogs fed a high protein diet (103 g/1000 kcal protein) at 50% MER to induce weight loss returned to weight and lean body mass levels similar to their preobesity values (30). Overweight dogs undergoing caloric restriction while being fed increasing levels of protein (approximately 57–111 g/1000 kcal) had less lean tissue loss compared to dogs eating the lower protein diets (31). The National Research Council daily recommended allowance of protein for dogs is $3.28 \, g/BW_{kg}^{0.75}$ and for cats is $4.96 \, g/BW_{kg}^{0.67}$ for maintenance (32). It has been recently suggested that $7.8 \, g/BW_{kg}^{0.75}$ is required to maintain lean body mass in cats (33). To ensure the diet chosen for the weight loss program will maintain adequate protein intake at the recommended level of caloric restriction, protein requirements should be calculated (Box 5.5).

(a)

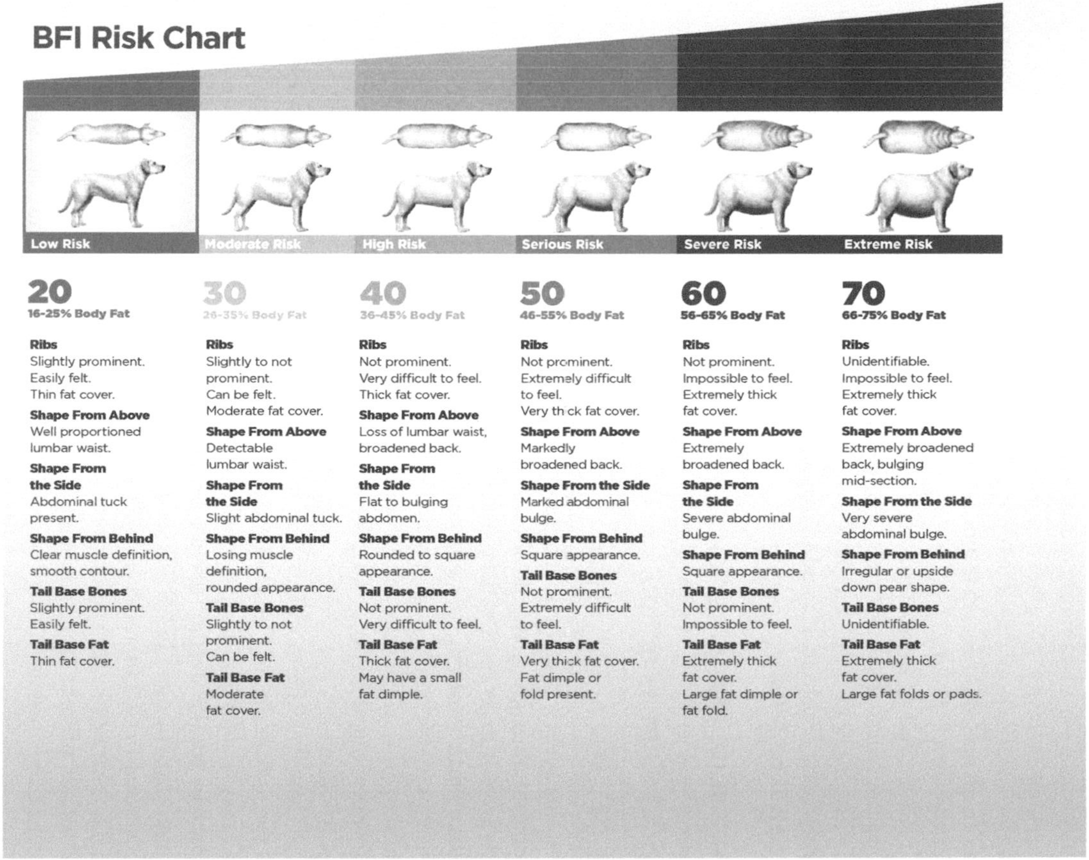

BFI Risk Chart

Low Risk	Moderate Risk	High Risk	Serious Risk	Severe Risk	Extreme Risk
20 16–25% Body Fat	**30** 26–35% Body Fat	**40** 36–45% Body Fat	**50** 46–55% Body Fat	**60** 56–65% Body Fat	**70** 66–75% Body Fat
Ribs Slightly prominent. Easily felt. Thin fat cover.	**Ribs** Slightly to not prominent. Can be felt. Moderate fat cover.	**Ribs** Not prominent. Very difficult to feel. Thick fat cover.	**Ribs** Not prominent. Extremely difficult to feel. Very thick fat cover.	**Ribs** Not prominent. Impossible to feel. Extremely thick fat cover.	**Ribs** Unidentifiable. Impossible to feel. Extremely thick fat cover.
Shape From Above Well proportioned lumbar waist.	**Shape From Above** Detectable lumbar waist.	**Shape From Above** Loss of lumbar waist, broadened back.	**Shape From Above** Markedly broadened back.	**Shape From Above** Extremely broadened back.	**Shape From Above** Extremely broadened back, bulging mid-section.
Shape From the Side Abdominal tuck present.	**Shape From the Side** Slight abdominal tuck.	**Shape From the Side** Flat to bulging abdomen.	**Shape From the Side** Marked abdominal bulge.	**Shape From the Side** Severe abdominal bulge.	**Shape From the Side** Very severe abdominal bulge.
Shape From Behind Clear muscle definition, smooth contour.	**Shape From Behind** Losing muscle definition, rounded appearance.	**Shape From Behind** Rounded to square appearance.	**Shape From Behind** Square appearance.	**Shape From Behind** Square appearance.	**Shape From Behind** Irregular or upside down pear shape.
Tail Base Bones Slightly prominent. Easily felt.	**Tail Base Bones** Slightly to not prominent. Can be felt.	**Tail Base Bones** Not prominent. Very difficult to feel.	**Tail Base Bones** Not prominent. Extremely difficult to feel.	**Tail Base Bones** Not prominent. Impossible to feel.	**Tail Base Bones** Unidentifiable.
Tail Base Fat Thin fat cover.	**Tail Base Fat** Moderate fat cover.	**Tail Base Fat** Thick fat cover. May have a small fat dimple.	**Tail Base Fat** Very thick fat cover. Fat dimple or fold present.	**Tail Base Fat** Extremely thick fat cover. Large fat dimple or fat fold.	**Tail Base Fat** Extremely thick fat cover. Large fat folds or pads.

(Continued)

Figure 5.2 **(a, b)** Canine and feline body fat index. (Reprinted with permission of Hill's Pet Nutrition, Inc.)

(b)

BFI Risk Chart

	Low Risk	Moderate Risk	High Risk	Serious Risk	Severe Risk	Extreme Risk
	20 16–25% Body Fat	**30** 26–35% Body Fat	**40** 36–45% Body Fat	**50** 46–55% Body Fat	**60** 56–65% Body Fat	**70** 66–75% Body Fat
Face	Minimal fat cover. Prominent bony structures.	Slight fat cover. Defined bony structures.	Slight to moderate fat cover. Defined to slight bony structures.	Moderate fat cover. Slight to minimal bony structures.	Thick fat cover. Minimal to no bony structures.	Very thick fat cover. No bony structures.
Head & Neck	Prominent distinction between head & shoulder. Loose scruff. No scruff fat.	Clear distinction between head & shoulder. Loose scruff. Slight scruff fat.	Clear to slight distinction between head & shoulder. Loose to snug scruff. Slight to moderate scruff fat.	Minimal distinction between head & shoulder. Loose to snug scruff. Moderate scruff fat.	Poor to no distinction between head & shoulder. Snug to tight scruff. Very thick scruff fat.	No distinction between head & shoulder. Tight scruff. Very thick scruff fat.
Sternum	Prominent. Very easy to palpate. Minimal pectoral fat.	Defined, slightly prominent. Easy to palpate. Slight to moderate pectoral fat.	Minimally prominent. Palpable. Moderate pectoral fat.	Poorly defined. Difficult to palpate. Thick pectoral fat.	Not prominent. Extremely difficult to palpate. Extremely thick pectoral fat.	Not prominent. Impossible to palpate. Extreme pectoral fat.
Scapula	Prominent. Very easy to palpate.	Defined, slightly prominent. Easy / very easy to palpate.	Slightly prominent. Easy to palpate.	Minimally to not prominent. Palpable.	Not prominent. Difficult to palpate.	Not prominent. Impossible to palpate.
Ribs	Prominent. Very easy to palpate.	Not prominent. Easy to palpate.	Not prominent. Palpable.	Not prominent. Difficult to palpate.	Not prominent. Extremely difficult to impossible to palpate.	Not prominent. Impossible to palpate.
Abdomen	Loose abdominal skin. Easy to palpate abdominal contents.	Loose abdominal skin with minimal fat. Easy to palpate abdominal contents.	Obvious skin fold with moderate fat. Easy to palpate abdominal contents.	Heavy fat pad. Difficult to palpate abdominal contents.	Very heavy fat pad, indistinct from abdominal fat. Impossible to palpate abdominal contents.	Extremely heavy fat pad, indistinct from abdominal fat. Impossible to palpate abdominal contents.
Tail Base	Prominent bony structure. Easy to palpate. Minimal fat cover.	Slightly to minimally prominent bony structure. Palpable. Slight fat cover.	Minimally prominent bony structure. Palpable. Slight to moderate fat cover.	Poorly defined bony structure. Difficult to palpate. Moderate to thick fat cover.	Bony structure not prominent. Very difficult to palpate. Very thick fat cover.	Bony structure not prominent. Extremely difficult to palpate. Extremely thick fat cover.
Shape From the Side	Moderate to slight abdominal tuck.	No abdominal tuck.	Slight abdominal bulge.	Moderate abdominal bulge.	Severe abdominal bulge.	Very severe abdominal bulge.
Shape From Above	Marked hourglass.	Slight hourglass / lumbar waist.	Lumbar waist.	Broadened back.	Severely broadened back.	Extremely broadened back.

Figure 5.2 (Continued)

BOX 5.1: Equations to estimate ideal body weight (11,12)

Equation 5.1:

$$\text{IBW (kg or lb)} = \frac{\text{Current body weight (kg or lb)} \times (100\% - \text{Current body fat \%})}{100\% - \text{Ideal body fat \%}}$$

Equation 5.2:

$$\text{IBW (kg or lb)} = \frac{\text{Current body weight (kg or lb)} \times (100\% - \% \text{ Excess body weight})}{100}$$

Equation 5.3:

$$\text{IBW (kg or lb)} = \frac{\text{Current body weight (kg or lb)} \times 100}{100 + (\text{Current BCS} - 5) \times 10}$$

Example: 10 yr female spayed (FS) Labrador retriever weighing 48 kg (105.6 lb), BCS 9/9, estimated 45% body fat

- Equation 5.1: 48 kg (105.6 lb) × (100% − 45%)/(100% − 20%) = 33 kg (72.6 lb)
- Equation 5.2: 48 kg (105.6 lb) × (100% − 40%)/100 = 28.8 kg (63.4 lb)
- Equation 5.3: 48 kg (105.6 lb) × 100/[100 + (9 − 5) × 10] = 34.3 kg (75.4 lb)

BOX 5.2: Predictive equation for body fat percentage (BF%) using morphometric measurements (8,9)

Dogs:

$$\text{BF\%} = 0.71 \times \text{Thoracic circumference} - 0.1 \times (\text{Pelvic circumference}/6)^2$$
$$- 5.78 \times \text{Hind limb length}^{0.8} + 26.56$$
$$\times (\text{Pelvic circumference}/\text{Head circumference}) + 2.06$$

Note: Measurements are in centimeters.

In addition to a high protein content, many therapeutic weight loss diets utilize a high fiber (HF) level to reduce caloric content and impart a satiety effect. A HF diet (92.5 g/1000 kcal total dietary fiber [TDF]) was associated with reduced caloric intake versus a lower fiber diet (39.1 g/1000 kcal TDF) in dogs. This effect was due to the reduced caloric density of the high versus low fiber diet (3138 kcal/kg vs. 3615 kcal/kg ME) rather than a change in volume intake (34). This effect was repeated when low and medium fiber diets were investigated, while reduced volume of food intake was also seen with diets high in crude fiber when fed an extra daily meal (35). When dogs were on an energy-restricted active weight loss program, there was no change in voluntary intake of an extra daily meal with TDF levels from 12.9 to 99.1 g/1000 kcal (36). Lean client-owned dogs have also been reported to receive more crude fiber than obese dogs, regardless of treats (37). Cats increase food intake to maintain similar total energy consumption when eating diets of varying fiber content (22–56 g/1000 kcal TDF), but cats eating HF diets consume a larger volume of food when offered an extra meal with a palatable, energy-dense diet (38). Other studies have shown decreased energy intake when cats are fed diets supplemented with kaolin or varying levels of cellulose, but diminished diet palatability may have been the main cause for these cats (39–41).

In dogs, a high protein–high fiber diet (HPHF; 103 g/1000 kcal protein, 60 g/1000 kcal crude fiber, 97 g/1000 kcal total dietary fiber, 2900 kcal/kg ME) was compared to a moderate protein–high fiber diet (MPHF; 86 g/1000 kcal protein, 87 g/1000 kcal crude fiber, 132 g/1000 kcal total dietary fiber, 2660 kcal/kg ME) and high protein–moderate fiber diet (HPMF; 104 g/1000 kcal protein, 35 g/1000 kcal crude fiber, 56 g/1000 kcal total dietary fiber, 3275 kcal/kg ME). HPHF dogs consumed less calories compared to HPMF and MPHF dogs (42). When fed an HPHF diet, overweight or obese dogs on an active weight loss program lost a greater percentage of weight (31.8% vs. 20.0%) at a faster rate (1.0%/week vs. 0.7%/week) than matched HPMF dogs. HPHF dogs also had a greater change in body fat mass loss compared with HPMF (58% vs. 37%) (43). When obese cats were fed canned or dry diets with 115–139 g/1000 kcal protein and 28–81 g/1000 kcal TDF as part of a controlled weight loss trial, body weight and BCS decreased similarly over time for all diets, but owners were least satisfied with and felt their cats were hungrier when fed only a dry diet with 115 g/1000 kcal protein and 81 g/1000 kcal TDF (26).

Rather than increasing the dietary fiber level, some weight loss feeding recommendations, especially for cats, utilize low carbohydrate (LC) diets. LC diets aim to put the body into a glycogenolytic state in which glycogen stores are depleted and the body moves toward lipolysis and β-oxidation as an alternative energy source. Increased acetyl-CoA production results in increased hepatic ketone body (acetone, acetoacetic acid, β-hydroxybutyric acid) production, providing an alternative energy source for most tissues and reserving glucose for glucose-dependent tissues such as brain and erythrocytes. The shift away from glucose results in decreased fasting and postprandial glucose and circulating insulin. These types of diets may have a metabolic advantage over HF diets, particularly in cats with obesity and insulin resistance that may result in diabetes mellitus (44), although weight loss regardless of diet selection is most important in controlling or achieving remission of diabetes mellitus in the cat (45).

Low fat diets are not specifically employed in canine or feline weight loss protocols. With the exception of LC diets, many canine and feline therapeutic diets do tend to utilize a lower fat content, however, as a means to achieve a reduced caloric density rather than due to a specific benefit of fat reduction.

5.3.1.2 DIET FORM AND ENERGY DENSITY

Diet selection should include consideration of the patient's preference (dry versus canned) and preference of the owner. Dry LC diets tend to be calorically dense when compared to HF therapeutic weight loss diets, and patient or owner adherence may

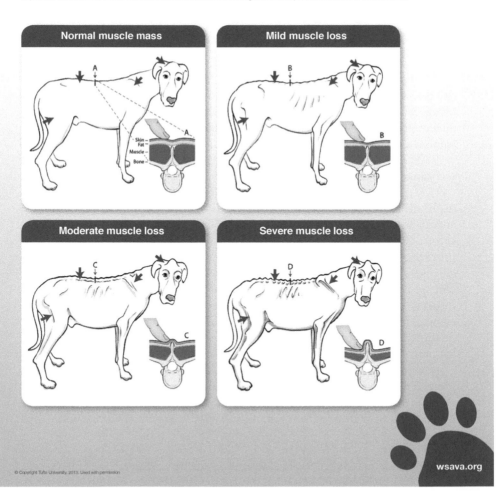

Figure 5.3 **(a, b)** Canine and feline muscle condition scoring system. (Global Nutrition Committee Toolkit provided courtesy of the World Small Animal Veterinary Association.) *(Continued)*

(b)

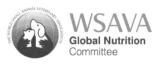

Muscle Condition Score

Muscle condition score is assessed by visualization and palpation of the spine, scapulae, skull, and wings of the ilia. Muscle loss is typically first noted in the epaxial muscles on each side of the spine; muscle loss at other sites can be more variable. Muscle condition score is graded as normal, mild loss, moderate loss, or severe loss. Note that animals can have significant muscle loss even if they are overweight (body condition score > 5/9). Conversely, animals can have a low body condition score (< 4/9) but have minimal muscle loss. Therefore, assessing both body condition score and muscle condition score on every animal at every visit is important. Palpation is especially important with mild muscle loss and in animals that are overweight. An example of each score is shown below.

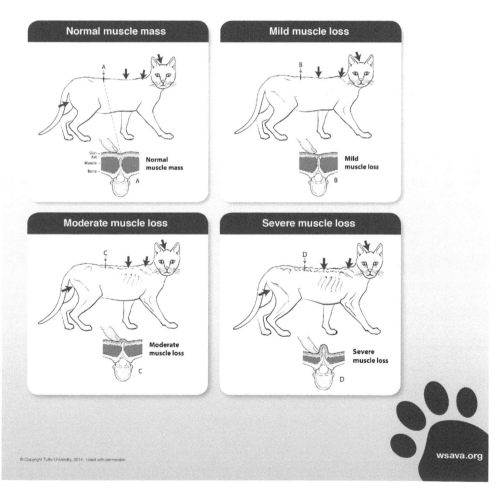

© Copyright Tufts University, 2014. Used with permission

wsava.org

Figure 5.3 (*Continued*)

BOX 5.3: Sources of caloric intake for companion animals

Primary diet: Commercial or home prepared
Commercial or home-prepared treats
Table scraps
Food for medication administration
Supplements
Wildlife
Feces
Trash
Food from other pets

BOX 5.4: Calculations for resting energy requirement (RER) and maintenance energy requirement (MER) for weight loss (11,21–23)

Calculation 1 (dogs and cats):
Resting energy requirement (RER):

- Exponential equation: $RER = (Body\ weight_{kg})^{0.75} \times 70$
- Linear equation: $RER = 30 \times (Body\ weight_{kg}) + 70$
  - Not for use in animals <2 kg or >25 kg

Maintenance energy requirement (MER):

- Dogs: $MER = RER \times 1.0$
- Cats: $MER = RER \times 0.8$

Calculation 2 (dogs only):
Option to adjust based on activity level:

- Inactive (<7250 steps/day): $MER = [(Body\ weight_{kg})^{0.75} \times 95] \times 0.45$
- Active (>7250 steps/day): $MER = [(Body\ weight_{kg})^{0.75} \times 95] \times 0.55$

Calculation 3 (dogs only):
Based on sex and neuter status:

- Neutered female: $MER = (Body\ weight_{kg})^{0.75} \times 60$
- Intact female: $MER = (Body\ weight_{kg})^{0.75} \times 70$
- Neutered male: $MER = (Body\ weight_{kg})^{0.75} \times 70$
- Intact male: $MER = (Body\ weight_{kg})^{0.75} \times 80$

Calculation 4 (cats only):

- $MER = (Body\ weight_{kg})^{0.711} \times 53$

Example: 5 yr FS beagle, estimated ideal weight 8.2 kg (18 lb), considered inactive

- Calculation 1: $8.2 \text{ kg}^{0.75} \times 70 = 339$ kcal $\times 1.0 = 339$ kcal/day
- Calculation 2: $8.2 \text{ kg}^{0.75} \times 95 = 460$ kcal $\times 0.45 = 207$ kcal/day
- Calculation 3: $8.2 \text{ kg}^{0.75} \times 60 = 291$ kcal/day

Example: 8 yr FS American domestic shorthair, estimated ideal weight 3.7 kg (8.14 lb)

- Calculation 1: $3.7 \text{ kg}^{0.75} \times 70 = 187$ kcal $\times 0.8 = 149$ kcal/day
- Calculation 4: $3.7 \text{ kg}^{0.711} \times 53 = 134$ kcal/day

be complicated by the small volume of food. For example, a cat with an IBW of 5 kg may need to consume 190 kcal per day for weight loss, which may be less than 1/3 standard 8-ounce measuring cup (approximately 45 grams kibble) of currently available therapeutic dry LC diets. Canned diets may increase satiety and weight loss in cats through higher moisture content. Energy intake and body weight were significantly decreased in cats consuming a canned diet compared to the same diet but with a lower moisture content (freeze-drying), suggesting that higher moisture foods may be of benefit versus dry foods during weight loss in cats (46).

Successful weight management can be achieved by both LC and HF diets, although there are limited studies comparing the success of weight management in cats consuming LC versus HF diets. Body condition and energy intake, not nutrient composition, influenced body weight during weight loss in one study (47). Another study evaluating owner-perceived satiety in cats undergoing weight loss

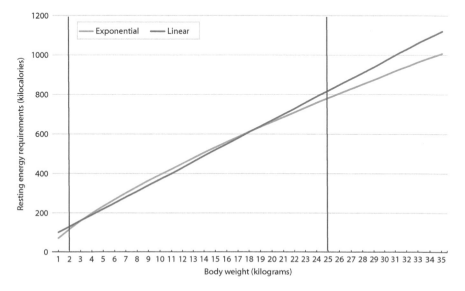

Figure 5.4 Exponential versus linear equation for calculation of resting energy requirements (RER).

BOX 5.5: Calculations for daily protein intake (32,33)

Calculation 1 (dogs):

Protein recommended allowance (RA) = 3.28 g/$BW_{kg}^{0.75}$

$$\text{Required dietary protein content} = \frac{\text{Protein RA}}{\text{Daily caloric intake}} \times 1000$$

Calculation 2 (cats):

Protein recommended allowance (RA) = 4.96 g/$BW_{kg}^{0.67}$

$$\text{Required dietary protein content} = \frac{\text{Protein RA}}{\text{Daily caloric intake}} \times 1000$$

Calculation 3 (cats):

Proposed protein requirement to maintain lean body mass = 7.8 g/$BW_{kg}^{0.75}$

$$\text{Required dietary protein content} = \frac{\text{Protein RA}}{\text{Daily caloric intake}} \times 1000$$

Example: 5 yr FS Beagle, estimated ideal weight 8.2 kg (18 lb), feeding 339 kcal/day

- Calculation 1:

$$8.2 \text{ kg}^{0.75} \times 3.28 = \frac{15.9 \text{ g protein}}{339 \text{ kcal}} \times 1000 = 46.9 \text{ g/1000 kcal protein}$$

Example: 8 yr FS American domestic shorthair, estimated ideal weight 3.7 kg (8.14 lb), feeding 149 kcal/day

- Calculation 2:

$$3.7 \text{ kg}^{0.67} \times 4.96 = \frac{11.9 \text{ g protein}}{149 \text{ kcal}} \times 1000 = 80 \text{ g/1000 kcal protein}$$

- Calculation 3:

$$3.7 \text{ kg}^{0.75} \times 7.8 = \frac{20.8 \text{ g protein}}{149 \text{ kcal}} \times 1000 = 140 \text{ g/1000 kcal protein}$$

---

was unable to find a difference between LC versus HF diets, although the sample size of this study was limited (48). If dry food is preferred, the authors typically recommend a high protein, low caloric density food (through added fiber and/or reduced fat), as LC diets tend to have higher fat levels, therefore a higher calorie density.

5.3.2 Portioning food for weight loss

Food for weight loss should be measured by weight, by portions of a can/pouch/tray, or with standard measuring cups. Measuring dry extruded kibble by weight is preferred, as use of measuring cups is associated with poor precision and accuracy (18% underestimate to an 80% overestimate in portion size), and accuracy is negatively associated with portion size (49). Dog owners are more likely to portion out a larger amount of kibble when using large bowls and large scoops as compared to small bowls and small scoops (50). It is possible owners using measuring cups, and certainly those using unmarked generic scoops, may be unintentionally providing a higher volume of food than intended, which will lead to inaccurate consumption reporting. Weighing food on a kitchen scale in grams is particularly useful in cats or small dogs in which there may be significant caloric differences as measuring cup volume changes. Calorie information as kcal/kg should be available on the individual product label or through the manufacturer. Switching to a smaller food bowl may also help some pet owners avoid the perception they are feeding smaller portions of food (50).

5.3.3 Setting treat guidelines

It is generally recommended that no more than 10% of total caloric intake come from food other than a complete and balanced diet for any pet to avoid dilution of nutrients with foods that are not complete and balanced. This includes treats, table food, foods for medication administration, and calories from supplements. Low calorie fruits and vegetables can be recommended to help owners maintain adherence to the feeding plan (Box 5.6). When selecting commercial treats, caloric content should be identified and restriction of the number of treats per day should be established. The use of a treat box or bag assembled daily for members of the household to dispense can be a useful feeding strategy to ensure overtreating does not occur. A daily treat allowance sheet may also help owners better utilize their treat allowances and avoid excess provisions (see Chapter 8, Appendix 8.3).

BOX 5.6: Low calorie fruits and vegetables for treat allowance (19)

Item	Common unit	1 cup (kcal)	100 grams (kcal)
Baby carrot, raw	1 large = 5 kcal		35
Green beans, raw	4" bean = 2 kcal	62	30
Bell pepper, green, raw	10 strips = 5 kcal	18	20
Celery, raw	5" stalk = 2 kcal	16	16
Zucchini, steamed/boiled, slices	1 medium = 33 kcal	28	15
Apple, with skin, raw	1 large = 116 kcal	65	52
Blueberries, raw	1 berry = 1 kcal	84	57
Watermelon, raw	1 ball = 4 kcal	46	30
Pumpkin, canned	1 tablespoon = 5 kcal	83	34

> ### BOX 5.7: Calculating rate of weight loss per week
>
> $$\text{Total rate of weight loss} = \frac{(\text{Previous weight} - \text{Current weight})}{\text{Previous weight}} \times 100$$
>
> $$\text{Weekly rate of weight loss} = \frac{\text{Total rate of weight loss}}{\#\,\text{Weeks since previous weight}}$$
>
> Example: 8 yr FS American domestic shorthair, previous weight 5 kg (11 lb), current weight 4.9 kg (10.8 lb), estimated ideal weight 3.7 kg (8.14 lb), 2 weeks since previous weight check
>
> - (5 kg − 4.9 kg)/5 kg × 100 = 2% total rate of weight loss
> - 2%/2 weeks = 1% loss per week

5.4 REEVALUATING THE WEIGHT LOSS PROGRAM

5.4.1 Routine follow-up

The initial weight loss visit should take place approximately 2–4 weeks after starting a weight loss regimen (see Chapter 8). At each visit, rate of weight loss (Box 5.7) is calculated, diet history since the start of the program reviewed, food intake adjusted, and potential adherence-related issues addressed. Additionally, BCS and evaluation of muscle condition score is assessed. A rate of weight loss between 1%–2% of body weight per week is recommended, but 0.5%–1% is acceptable in cats. If the patient is within this acceptable range, no changes to the diet plan are made unless the owner reports potential adherence-related issues.

For patients whose rate is outside this acceptable range or who are having adherence-related issues, a detailed review of the patient's current intake should be compared to the recommended weight loss program. Separated feeding of pets needs to be reemphasized and the owner should be asked to list exactly what foods are being fed, the volume or weight of each item, and if any other household members may be feeding outside of the diet plan. This review will likely identify behavioral modifications that can be addressed (see Chapter 6). If the rate of weight loss is outside the acceptable range and no adherence issues are identified, the food intake is adjusted accordingly. Calories are generally reduced by 5%–10% (including treats), and weight rechecks are continued every 2–4 weeks until consistent weight loss occurs. With patients experiencing good weight loss progress, longer intervals between weight rechecks can be considered, but monthly weigh-ins are preferred.

5.4.2 Long-term success

Depending on the degree of obesity, successful and safe weight loss may take several months and potentially over a year. Over 12 weeks, only 0.6% of dogs maintained a rate of weight loss >2% per week with an average of $0.9 \pm 0.45\%$ of initial body weight per week. Rates of weight loss also declined from an average of 1.3% per week to 0.8% per week over the same time frame (22). In a similar study, cats lost $0.8 \pm 0.50\%$ of initial body weight per week and declined from 1.2% per week to 0.7% per week (23).

Once the IBW or TBW is achieved, caloric intake can be adjusted to maintain the current body weight. Dogs have a maintenance energy requirement of 52–104 kcal/$kg^{0.75}$ following weight loss, typically only approximately 10% more than that required during weight loss (51). Although similar data has not been published in cats, a caloric increase of no more than 10% is recommended for weight maintenance in both cats and dogs. Additional follow-up (usually one to three rechecks) is needed after maintenance feeding adjustments to ensure ideal/target weight is maintained. If given free choice access to food after successfully losing weight, dogs regain weight (52). Dogs will also achieve the same level of obesity faster and with less calories than they needed to originally become obese (53).

Dogs switched to a standard maintenance diet consume more calories and regain more weight, suggesting long-term feeding of purpose formulated weight management diets can significantly limit regain (54). Forty-nine percent of previously obese dogs and 46% of previously obese cats that achieved ideal or target body weight gained more than 5% of body weight back (54,55). Cats that rebound are more likely to regain over 50% of their original weight loss when compared to dogs. While these data may be discouraging, it is important to keep in mind that the majority (51%–54%) of dogs and cats maintain or continue to lose weight after a successful weight loss program.

5.5 CONCLUSIONS

Although obstacles encountered during a weight loss plan can be discouraging, it is important to remind owners it can be done as long as they are willing to put in the necessary time and dedication required to maintain long-term weight success. Long-term continuation of a weight management diet with a low caloric density, specific treat allowance, and exercise are recommended to avoid relapse of weight gain.

REFERENCES

1. Lund EM, Armstrong PJ, Kirk CA, Klausner JS. Prevalence and risk factors for obesity in adult cats from private US veterinary practices. *The International Journal of Applied Research in Veterinary Medicine* 2005;3:88–96.
2. Lund EM, Armstrong PJ, Kirk CA, Klausner JS. Prevalence and risk factors for obesity in adult dogs from private US veterinary practices. *The International Journal of Applied Research in Veterinary Medicine* 2006;4:177–186.
3. Rohlf VI, Toukhsati S, Coleman GJ, Bennett PC. Dog obesity: Can dog caregivers' (owners') feeding and exercise intentions and behaviors be predicted from attitudes? *Journal of Applied Animal Welfare Science* 2010;13:213–236.

4. White GA, Hobson-West P, Cobb K, Craigon J, Hammond R, Millar KM. Canine obesity: Is there a difference between veterinarian and owner perception? *Journal of Small Animal Practice* 2011;52:622–626.
5. Rowe EC, Browne WJ, Casey RA, Gruffydd-Jones TJ, Murray JK. Early-life risk factors identified for owner-reported feline overweight and obesity at around two years of age. *Preventive Veterinary Medicine* 2017;14:39–48.
6. Laflamme D. Development and validation of a body condition score system for cats: A clinical tool. *Feline Practice* 1997;25:13–17.
7. Laflamme D. Development and validation of a body condition score system for dogs. *Canine Practice* 1997;22:10–15.
8. Witzel AL, Kirk CA, Henry GA, Toll PW, Brejda JJ, Paetau-Robinson I. Use of a novel morphometric method and body fat index system for estimation of body composition in overweight and obese dogs. *Journal of the American Veterinary Medical Association* 2014;22:1279–1284.
9. Witzel AL, Kirk CA, Henry GA, Toll PW, Brejda JJ, Paetau-Robinson I. Use of a morphometric method and body fat index system for estimation of body composition in overweight and obese cats. *Journal of the American Veterinary Medical Association* 2014;24:1285–1290.
10. Mawby DI, Bartges JW, d'Avignon A, Laflamme DP, Moyers TD, Cottrell T. Comparison of various methods for estimating body fat in dogs. *Journal of the American Animal Hospital Association* 2004;40:109–114.
11. Brooks D, Churchill J, Fein K et al. 2014 AAHA weight management guidelines for dogs and cats. *Journal of the American Animal Hospital Association* 2014;50:1–11.
12. German AJ, Holden SL, Bissot T, Morris PJ, Biourge V. Use of starting condition score to estimate changes in body weight and composition during weight loss in obese dogs. *Research in Veterinary Science* 2009;87:249–254.
13. Bjornvad CR, Nielsen DH, Armstrong PJ et al. Evaluation of a nine-point body condition scoring system in physically inactive pet cats. *American Journal of Veterinary Research* 2011;72:433–437.
14. Freeman LM. Cachexia and sarcopenia: Emerging syndromes of importance in dogs and cats. *Journal of Veterinary Internal Medicine* 2012;26:3–17.
15. Hutchinson D, Sutherland-Smith J, Watson AL, Freeman LM. Assessment of methods of evaluating sarcopenia in old dogs. *American Journal of Veterinary Research* 2012;73:1794–800.
16. Freeman L, Becvarova I, Cave N et al. WSAVA Nutritional Assessment Guidelines. *Journal of Small Animal Practice* 2011;52:385–396.
17. Michel KE, Anderson W, Cupp C, Laflamme DP. Correlation of a feline muscle mass score with body composition determined by dual-energy x-ray absorptiometry. *British Journal of Nutrition* 2011;10:S57–S59.
18. AAFCO. *2018 Official Publication of the Association of American Feed Control Officials.* 2018.

19. United States Department of Agriculture Agricultural Research Service. *USDA Food Composition Database*. Available from: https://ndb.nal.usda.gov/ndb/.

20. German AJ, Holden SL, Gernon LJ, Morris PJ, Biourge V. Do feeding practices of obese dogs, before weight loss, affect the success of weight management? *British Journal of Nutrition* 2011;10:S97–S100.

21. Wakshlag JJ, Struble AM, Warren BS et al. Evaluation of dietary energy intake and physical activity in dogs undergoing a controlled weight-loss program. *Journal of the American Veterinary Medical Association* 2012;24:413–419.

22. Flanagan J, Bissot T, Hours M-A, Moreno B, Feugier A, German AJ. Success of a weight loss plan for overweight dogs: The results of an international weight loss study. *PLOS ONE* 2017;12:e0184199.

23. Flanagan J, Bissot T, Hours M-A, Moreno B, German AJ. An international multi-centre cohort study of weight loss in overweight cats: Differences in outcome in different geographical locations. *PLOS ONE* 2018;13:e0200414.

24. Linder DE, Freeman LM, Morris P et al. Theoretical evaluation of risk for nutritional deficiency with caloric restriction in dogs. *Veterinary Quarterly* 2012;32:123–129.

25. Linder DE, Freeman LM, Holden SL, Biourge V, German AJ. Status of selected nutrients in obese dogs undergoing caloric restriction. *BMC Veterinary Research* 2013;9:19.

26. Bissot T, Servet E, Vidal S et al. Novel dietary strategies can improve the outcome of weight loss programmes in obese client-owned cats. *Journal of Feline Medicine and Surgery* 2010;12:104–112.

27. Levine ED, Erb HN, Schoenherr B, Houpt KA. Owner's perception of changes in behaviors associated with dieting in fat cats. *Journal of Veterinary Behavior: Clinical Applications and Research* 2016;11:37–41.

28. Westerterp-Plantenga MS, Nieuwenhuizen A, Tomé D, Soenen S, Westerterp KR. Dietary protein, weight loss, and weight maintenance. *Annual Review of Nutrition* 2009;29:21–41.

29. Westerterp-Plantenga MS, Lemmens SG, Westerterp KR. Dietary protein: Its role in satiety, energetics, weight loss and health. *British Journal of Nutrition* 2012;10:S105–S112.

30. Blanchard G, Nguyen P, Gayet C, Leriche I, Siliart B, Paragon B-M. Rapid weight loss with a high-protein low-energy diet allows the recovery of ideal body composition and insulin sensitivity in obese dogs. *Journal of Nutrition* 2004;13:2148S–2150S.

31. Hannah SS, Laflamme DP. Increased dietary protein spares lean body mass during weight loss in dogs [Abstract]. *Journal of Veterinary Internal Medicine* 1998;12:224.

32. National Research Council of the National Academies. Nutrient requirements and dietary nutrient concentrations. In: *Nutrient Requirements of Dogs and Cats*. Washington, DC: National Academies Press; 2006, pp. 354–370.

33. Laflamme DP, Hannah SS. Increased dietary protein promotes fat loss and reduces loss of lean body mass during weight loss in cats. *The International Journal of Applied Research in Veterinary Medicine* 2005;5:2–68.
34. Jackson JR, Laflamme DP, Owens SF. Effects of dietary fiber content on satiety in dogs. *Veterinary Clinical Nutrition* 1997;4:130–134.
35. Jewell DE, Toll PW. Effects of fiber on food intake in dogs. *Veterinary Clinical Nutrition* 1996;3:115–118.
36. Butterwick RF, Markwell PJ. Effect of amount and type of dietary fiber on food intake in energy-restricted dogs. *American Journal of Veterinary Research* 1997;58:272–276.
37. Heuberger R, Wakshlag J. The relationship of feeding patterns and obesity in dogs. *Journal of Animal Physiology and Animal Nutrition* 2011;95:98–105.
38. Loureiro BA, Sakomura NK, Vasconcellos RS et al. Insoluble fibres, satiety and food intake in cats fed kibble diets. *Journal of Animal Physiology and Animal Nutrition* 2017;10:824–834.
39. Kanarek RB. Availability and caloric density of the diet as determinants of meal patterns in cats. *Physiology & Behavior* 1975;15:611–618.
40. Prola L, Dobenecker B, Kienzle E. Interaction between dietary cellulose content and food intake in cats. *Journal of Nutrition* 2006;13:1988S–1990S.
41. Hirsch E, Dubose C, Jacobs HL. Dietary control of food intake in cats. *Physiology & Behavior* 1978;20:287–295.
42. Weber M, Bissot T, Servet E, Sergheraert R, Biourge V, German AJ. A high-protein, high-fiber diet designed for weight loss improves satiety in dogs. *Journal of Veterinary Internal Medicine* 2007;21:1203–1208.
43. German AJ, Holden SL, Bissot T, Morris PJ, Biourge V. A high protein high fibre diet improves weight loss in obese dogs. *Veterinary Journal* 2010;18:294–297.
44. Bennett N, Greco DS, Peterson ME, Kirk C, Mathes M, Fettman MJ. Comparison of a low carbohydrate-low fiber diet and a moderate carbohydrate-high fiber diet in the management of feline diabetes mellitus. *Journal of Feline Medicine and Surgery* 2006;8:73–84.
45. Hoenig M, Thomaseth K, Waldron M, Ferguson DC. Insulin sensitivity, fat distribution, and adipocytokine response to different diets in lean and obese cats before and after weight loss. *American Journal of Physiology: Regulatory, Integrative and Comparative Physiology* 2007;29:R227–R234.
46. Wei A, Fascetti AJ, Villaverde C, Wong RK, Ramsey JJ. Effect of water content in a canned food on voluntary food intake and body weight in cats. *American Journal of Veterinary Research* 2011;72:918–923.
47. Michel KE, Bader A, Shofer FS, Barbera C, Oakley DA, Giger U. Impact of time-limited feeding and dietary carbohydrate content on weight loss in group-housed cats. *Journal of Feline Medicine and Surgery* 2005;7:49–55.
48. Cline M, Witzel A, Moyers T, Kirk C. Comparison of high fiber and low carbohydrate diet on owner-perceived satiety of cats during weight loss. *Am J Anim Vet Sci* 2012;7:18–25.

49. German AJ, Holden SL, Mason SL et al. Imprecision when using measuring cups to weigh out extruded dry kibbled food. *Journal of Animal Physiology and Animal Nutrition* 2011;95:368–373.

50. Murphy M, Lusby AL, Bartges JW, Kirk CA. Size of food bowl and scoop affects amount of food owners feed their dogs. *Journal of Animal Physiology and Animal Nutrition* 2012;96:237–241.

51. German AJ, Holden SL, Mather NJ, Morris PJ, Biourge V. Low-maintenance energy requirements of obese dogs after weight loss. *British Journal of Nutrition* 2011;10:S93–S96.

52. Laflamme D, Kuhlman G. The effect of weight-loss regimen on subsequent weight maintenance in dogs. *Nutrition Research* 1995;15:1019–1028.

53. Nagaoka D, Mitsuhashi Y, Angell R, Bigley KE, Bauer JE. Re-induction of obese body weight occurs more rapidly and at lower caloric intake in beagles. *Journal of Animal Physiology and Animal Nutrition* 2010;94:287–292.

54. German AJ, Holden SL, Morris PJ, Biourge V. Long-term follow-up after weight management in obese dogs: The role of diet in preventing regain. *Veterinary Journal* 2012;19:65–70.

55. Deagle G, Holden SL, Biourge V, Morris PJ, German AJ. Long-term follow-up after weight management in obese cats. *Journal of Nutritional Science* 2014;3:e25.

6

Behavioral management of obesity

DEBORAH E. LINDER AND MEGAN K. MUELLER

6.1 INTRODUCTION

Obesity is a complex nutritional disorder that often requires comprehensive management beyond a standard diet and exercise program and includes incorporation of an understanding of human–animal interaction to be successful. Effective client communication can assist the veterinary team in appreciating each family's unique relationship with the pets in the household and keep the human–animal bond intact. Thus, obesity treatment can be multimodal and include management from both medical and psychological perspectives to achieve success in behavioral management. Though obesity can be a challenging disorder to manage over the life of a pet, veterinarians can go beyond standard treatment to incorporate the unique relationship between the pet owner and pet into the plan. This not only strengthens the bond between owners and their pets, but can also lead to increased overall success in obesity treatment.

6.2 THE IMPACT OF OWNER PERCEPTION ON BEHAVIOR AND OBESITY

Risk factors for pet obesity vary in studies conducted worldwide on dogs and cats (1–8). Owner-related factors in one epidemiologic study were almost exclusively found as risk factors for obesity (3). This included owner age and behaviors controlled by owners, such as frequency of treats and amount of exercise. Many owner-related and behavioral risk factors for obesity highlight the need for veterinarians to fully understand the behaviors of the pet and the owner, as well as how the family dynamics and the pet–owner relationship may affect weight status and effectiveness of interventions (Table 6.1).

6.2.1 Perception of obesity

One notable risk factor for obesity is the pet owner's underestimation of the pet's body condition score (BCS). In two separate studies, 39% of owners underestimated their pet's BCS, even after knowing their pet's BCS as assessed by a veterinarian or trained assessor in some instances (9,10). Further evidence of misperception of ideal body weight among pet owners is highlighted by Bland and colleagues (11), in which half of the owners who "correctly" identified their pets' BCS score at more than ideal weight still did not consider their pet to be overweight. Figure 6.1 highlights opportunities for veterinary hospitals to address this discrepancy by pairing BCS charts with weight scales in waiting rooms. This discrepancy between owner and veterinarian views of an ideal body condition may stem from public perception that an overweight condition is the standard of beauty. For example, one study on show dogs revealed that almost 1 in every

Table 6.1 Owner-related risk factors for pet obesity

Feeding table scraps
Feeding snacks and treats
Increased owner age
Decreased owner income
Decreased dog exercise
Owner knowledge of pet body condition

Source: Courcier EA et al., *Journal of Small Animal Practice* 2010;51:362–367; Rohlf VI et al., *Journal of Applied Animal Welfare Science* 2010;13:213–236; White GA et al., *Journal of Small Animal Practice* 2011;52:622–626; Bland IM et al., *Preventative Veterinary Medicine* 2009;92:333–340.

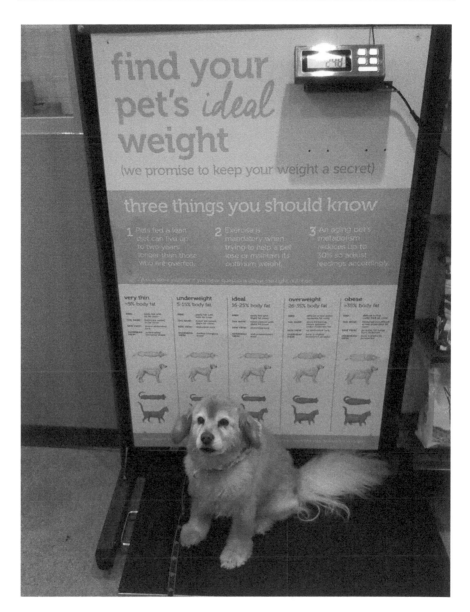

Figure 6.1 Incorporation of a body condition scoring chart with a weight scale in a veterinary hospital to encourage conversation about ideal body condition.

5 show dogs was overweight (12), and similar findings have been described in show cats as well (13). Owner perception can also affect behavior of pet owners and their adherence to weight management plans. For example, when considering feeding behaviors, studies have shown that the size of the food bowl and food scoop affects the amount of food owners feed their dogs (14). Furthermore, even veterinary staff's accuracy on feeding amounts varied from an 18% underestimate to an 80%

overestimate of the intended amount (15). With many owner-related behavioral risk factors for obesity combined with a misperception of body condition and feeding practices, weight management in pets requires comprehensive treatment that includes the owner and pet behavior and extends beyond the standard diet and exercise regimen.

6.2.2 Understanding owner perceptions

When discussing obesity with owners and gathering information as part of a complete diet history, taking time to fully understand the environment and behaviors of pets and pet owners will allow for assessment of the owner's readiness to change and ability to commit to a weight management plan. Some pet owners may not be ready to make behavioral changes necessary for weight loss and are still contemplating weight management for their pet. In these situations, client education and monitoring may be the best course of action before engaging in a comprehensive program requiring change from the pet owner. However, those owners who are prepared for or already taking action for weight management for their pet would best benefit from specific individualized plans and feedback. For example, pet owners may think that they just need to pick a "diet food," but are not sure which diet to select or are unaware they may need to change their behaviors for how they provide treats outside the main diet. Providing vague directions, such as "switch to a light food" or "cut back a little on the kibble," is not effective and can increase confusion for pet owners, while not addressing how behaviors such as excess provision of treats, and therefore calories, contribute to obesity (16).

Engaging pet owners and understanding their perceptions of weight-related issues and nutrition for their pets can provide veterinarians with an idea of the pet owners' readiness to change, which can impact the plan and behavioral changes that are suggested. Guidance on assessing readiness to change has been described elsewhere (17). Although initiating the conversation with owners about their pets' weight can be challenging, understanding the pet owner's perspective can guide management, and talking tips have been described to assist the veterinary health care team in these discussions (18).

Through these discussions, owners may relay that they would be interested in pursuing any plan that the veterinarian recommends, or they may explain their level or ability of commitment, which could guide weight management and behavioral recommendations. For owners interested in any type of plan, veterinarians can focus solely on medical factors that guide management, such as diet selection based on nutrient needs of the patient or starting calorie intake. However, in other instances, veterinarians may need to balance medical and social or psychological factors to develop a weight management plan to ensure success. For example, a pet owner's work schedule and feeding behaviors may need to be considered in dietary selection and obesity treatment. If a dog can only be taken out for a walk twice a day due to an owner's work schedule, a higher fiber diet that results in increased fecal output may not be ideal for that situation. In this case, though fiber may help some pets feel more satiated, if this were recommended to an owner without considering their feeding behaviors, pet owners may quit the program due to their pet defecating in the house and decide weight management is too difficult. Needs of other pets in the household may also need to be considered for similar logistics to ensure adherence. By understanding clients' backgrounds and perspectives, weight management and in particular behavioral change can be approached by the veterinarian in a way that clients will accept and engage in for optimal success.

6.3 INTEGRATING PSYCHOLOGY AND BEHAVIORAL MANAGEMENT INTO OBESITY TREATMENT

An important facet of successful weight management is the role that human–animal relationships can play in obesity prevention and treatment. Owners may need social and psychological support in addition to medical support as they implement weight management plans. Understanding the dynamics of human–animal relationships can be useful for practitioners in developing successful treatment plans with their clients. This section will discuss the process of putting social science theory into practice with practical management examples of the psychosocial aspects of a weight management program being incorporated into standard nutritional management.

6.3.1 The discussion of pet obesity

Veterinarians who are uncomfortable having a conversation about obesity are not alone, because communication about weight management is also a hesitation for many human health care providers (19). Human obesity and its related comorbidities represent a serious public health concern that parallels pet obesity, with a tripling of human obesity incidence in the past 30 years (20). Similar to veterinary medicine, the development of effective and maintainable interventions to treat obesity remains both a priority and a challenge in human medicine. Human health care providers and veterinarians share further challenges in that the approach to each patient or client may need to be individualized to their needs. In veterinary medicine, it can be helpful to base this approach on the owners' behaviors and relationships with their pets as a part of prioritizing a conversation about weight management. Three scenarios are included here, which have been discussed in detail elsewhere (18).

6.3.1.1 INFORMATION-BASED EXAMPLE

In the authors' experience, some pet owners have been upset that no one had previously mentioned their pets' weight as a potential health risk. This then led to the assumption that their pets were an ideal or healthy weight based on their veterinarians' lack of concern. This topic can be broached by asking whether anyone has ever discussed the pet's weight before. A discussion of health consequences, such as the risk of diabetes mellitus in overweight cats, can also be included. This can then be a casual start to a conversation that normalizes the condition and addresses health information in a neutral way without inciting blame or emotion, which owners may respond to favorably.

6.3.1.2 COMPARATIVE EXAMPLE

Owners who are also overweight often bring up similar struggles they are experiencing with obesity once the topic is introduced for their pet. Although it is not within veterinary ethics for veterinarians to provide weight management advice for humans, drawing on similarities may prove helpful for discussion purposes. An example noted in one review provides guidance if an owner were to say, "I know I'd rather have a cookie than kibble," a potential response could be, "In moderation, treats are fine, but, just like us, our pets could get sick if they ate only candy or cookies all the time. Would you like to discuss a possible weight management plan that includes balanced food and treats that your pet likes?" (18).

6.3.1.3 EMOTIONAL EXAMPLE

Some pet owners have a strong emotional attachment to their pets, and their behaviors regarding their pets reflect that strong bond. For example, more than half of pet owners say that their animals are allowed to sleep in their beds, and many pet owners anecdotally note that they buy their pets presents, cook meals for them, and dress them up, engaging in numerous anthropomorphic behaviors (21). Emotion can be a barrier to engaging in weight loss with examples in client statements such as, "It's cruel to 'starve' my pet and not give him what he wants." These emotional statements can be addressed or even used in a positive manner with an explanation of the impact of weight loss. For example, conversations can start that explain that weight loss is not harmful to pets and does not cause them pain. The opposite is actually true: Overweight pets are more likely to be in pain and can have worse quality of life such as decreased vitality (22). Weight loss does not hurt them but in fact makes them feel better. Further, a discussion that pets who "beg" may just be trained to go to their owners as providers of food, can be used to introduce the concept of food dispensing toys or automatic feeders to reduce food-seeking behaviors, as seen in Figure 6.2.

6.3.2 Incorporating perception in the initial weight discussion

In the authors' clinical experience, the emotional example is a very common exam room encounter and can sometimes be the most challenging to address given some clients' strongly held beliefs and prior perception of weight management. It has been shown that pet owners' perception of guilt or fear of depriving their pet is used as rationale for not engaging in weight loss plans (11). However, data now support that this line of thinking may be a misperception that should be discussed with pet owners and discussion may increase owner engagement in behavior change (22). For example, one study has shown that pets have a decreased quality of life when overweight and improve in these measures (such as vitality and pain) after successful weight loss (22). Discussing the quality-of-life consequences of obesity and the benefits of weight loss may help alleviate owner hesitancy from misperceptions of guilt. In addition, although pet owners may find it challenging to associate current obesity with clinical disease repercussions in the future, veterinarians can emphasize effects on a pet's current quality of

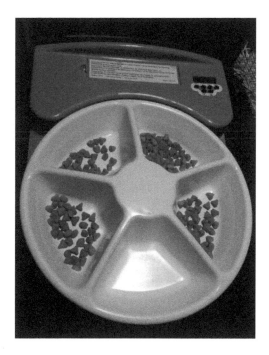

Figure 6.2 One example of an automatic food dispenser that can be set to provide timed, measured feeding portions to pets (5-Meal Automatic Pet Feeder by PetSafe[R]).

life that may be adversely affected by obesity to create the need for urgency in behavior change. A validated quality-of-life questionnaire can be used with pet owners to objectively measure these effects and how they change over time with weight management (22). When initiating and implementing weight management plans, a discussion that focuses on common goals shared by the veterinarian and the owner, namely, the well-being and comfort of the pet, can help to ease owners into the conversation and address the root of obesogenic behaviors.

6.4 CREATING EFFECTIVE WEIGHT MANAGEMENT PLANS BY ADDRESSING EMOTIONAL BEHAVIORS

Pet ownership and a strong bond between pets and their owners has been associated with may beneficial human mental health outcomes (23). The benefits of simply interacting with animals can include increased empathy (24), a sense of emotional support (25), and reduced loneliness (26) and stress (27). Since owners can have such profound relationships with their pets that their mental health is positively affected, weight management programs that affect this connection must be tailored to preserve this relationship to ensure adherence and success in weight loss. Understanding pet owners' behaviors and attachment to their pets helps to build trust between the veterinarians and pet owners. Building on this trust, weight management plans can be created together with veterinarians and pet owners in a way that reinforces owners' relationship with their pets and does not threaten that beneficial bond.

Interestingly, strong feelings of attachment may affect what behaviors pet owners are willing to change, influencing treatment in both positive and negative ways. For example, owners who are highly bonded to their pets may be more willing to devote financial resources and time to obtaining veterinary care and seeking weight management plans. However, high levels of attachment may also be associated with emotional dependency and obesogenic behaviors, such as some owners in clinical experience who provide an excess of food (and calories) to show love and affection to their pet. An owner who has a strong emotional relationship with an animal may be less inclined to change feeding behaviors, such as providing high calorie treats, because those behaviors represent a part of that relationship. For example, when engaging pet owners in a dietary history, it may be helpful to ask them to describe their daily routine with their pet, which would provide open-ended answers. Further questioning such as, "Which of those activities do you feel strongly about including in our weight loss plan?" will elicit behaviors that pet owners feel are critical to their bond with their pet and may sabotage weight loss plans if not incorporated in some way.

In the authors' experience, these questions can often reveal nonnegotiables that can be incorporated to increase adherence to weight management plans. For example, if an owner says that every night the pet needs to have a chew treat while the owner watches TV, a less calorically dense substitute for that treat can be made in order to preserve that aspect of their relationship while adhering to a weight management plan. This way, the owner still gets to engage in the desired behavior (providing a special food item and spending time with their pet), but the treat itself or the calories in the treat can be altered without adversely affecting their relationship. In another scenario, an owner who notes that it may be emotionally challenging to initiate exercise with a pet that does not seem to enjoy physical activity can be redirected to pair feeding time with exercise in a way that the pet and the pet owner can both derive pleasure. For example, instead of putting food into a bowl, pieces of a dry kibble could be distributed throughout the house or used in a game of fetch for cats or dogs. In cases such as these, an understanding of the emotional attachment between the owner and pet can help veterinarians and owners devise ways to address challenges and still be successful in weight loss.

6.5 CONSIDERING THE ROLE OF FAMILY DYNAMICS IN BEHAVIORAL MANAGEMENT OF OBESITY

Understanding human–animal relationships in different family settings can help veterinarians develop programs and behavior changes that are feasible to implement within the existing family dynamics. When collecting a diet history and discussing the potential plan, owners should also be asked about other members of the family and their relationships with the pet. It can be useful to ask clients specific questions about which family member(s) are responsible for various aspects of the pet's care such as feeding, exercise, and grooming

Table 6.2 Behavior-related example questions to include in a dietary history

Do any pets have access to other pets' food?
How many people live in your household?
Who in the family feeds your pet?
How does your family decide how much to feed your pet?
Describe mealtime for your pet.
Does your pet beg? If so, please describe the behavior.

(Table 6.2). This information guides development of a weight management plan that fits into the existing family structure and capitalizes on relationships that already exist. In addition, discussing family human–animal relationships can assist in preemptively addressing any potential barriers to weight management plan adherence. For example, in multiperson households, an accurate diet history can sometimes only be obtained after asking the entire family for a description of how the pet is fed. In the authors' experience, members of the household may not be aware of food items provided to their pet(s) by others in the household. Sometimes these feeding behaviors are kept hidden on purpose from others in the household, while in other cases, pet owners just may not communicate on every food item given to their pet(s).

In either of these scenarios, an effective method to address feeding habits of multiple owners is to discuss a daily feeding schedule when all family members are present. This can include the daily portions of the intended complete and balanced food, as well as various treats within the designated calories of a treat allowance. In order to ensure that pets are not accidentally fed multiple times or fed more than this designated amount, a food box allowance can be prepared nightly by the family for the following day that includes a variety of treats and meals adding up to the desired calorie amount. In this situation, everyone in the family can see for themselves that their pet does indeed receive a lot of treats and food throughout the day; it is simply spread out among many family members. This time spent creating a food box allowance together as a family can also increase time for communication among family members, and anecdotally in clients, this has allowed for a strengthening of the bond between family members and pets. Addressing the needs of all family members within a household can minimize adherence concerns and increase success and enjoyment in implementing the weight management plan.

6.6 PAIRING PET AND OWNER BEHAVIOR FOR MUTUAL SUCCESS

Although the majority of behavioral management focuses on adjustment of behaviors to benefit the health and weight status of pets, the benefits of the human–animal bond can also be harnessed for physical health benefits in humans as well. One study (28) has shown that engaging in a weight loss program for pets can have a positive impact on pet owners' physical health and activity level. In addition, overweight pet owners may have a stronger attachment to their pets and have less perceived social support from peers than healthy-weight pet owners (29). If overweight owners are indeed looking to their pets for social support instead of their human contemporaries, engaging pet owners in behaviors that could benefit themselves as well as their pet can be particularly helpful and increase chances for success. Regardless of weight status, however, all pet owners could improve their relationship with their pets through healthy behaviors such as exercise instead of through provision of extra calories in treats, which is how some owners express their love. Figure 6.3 highlights an opportunity for pets and owners to engage in physical activity such as walking or swimming together.

Future research into integrative treatment programs is warranted to target human and animal health. Family-oriented obesity treatment programs in which overweight families and their pets can become healthy together could have immense potential for significantly affecting health and wellness in veterinary and human medicine. Until further research is conducted on the most effective methodology for this type of a program, veterinarians should focus on preserving beneficial healthy human–animal relationships. This is best done by understanding the bonds between owners and pets, fostering healthy behaviors already present, and creating healthy alternatives and substitutes for behaviors that predispose both people and their pets to obesity without sacrificing beneficial human–animal relationships and bonds.

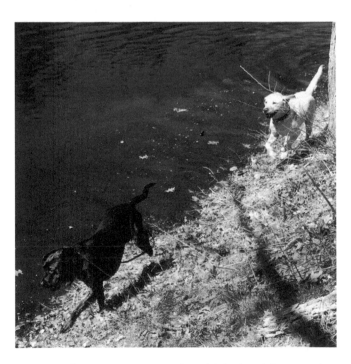

Figure 6.3 Dogs and pet owners can enjoy physical activity together such as walking and swimming together.

6.7 CONCLUSION

Many risk factors, combined with the complexity humans can have in their relationships with pets, can create an environment conducive to pet obesity. On the positive side, integrating the many medical and social science aspects of obesity can improve success in weight management. Although treatment of obesity can be intensive and require comprehensive management, there are many novel aspects of obesity treatment, even many yet to be investigated, that can lead to a rewarding and enjoyable owner, pet, and veterinarian experience. Weight management plans that take a comprehensive approach include understanding and integration of the complex relationship owners have with their pets, which extend beyond standard nutritional management and improve success.

REFERENCES

1. McGreevy PD, Thomson PC, Pride C, Fawcett A, Grassi T, Jones B. Prevalence of obesity in dogs examined by Australian veterinary practices and the risk factors involved. *Veterinary Record* 2005;156:695–702.
2. Lund EM, Armstrong PJ, Kirk CA, Klausner JS. Prevalence and risk factors for obesity in adult dogs from private US veterinary practices. *International Journal of Applied Research in Veterinary Medicine* 2006;4:177–186.
3. Courcier EA, Thomson RM, Mellor DJ, Yam PS. An epidemiological study of environmental factors associated with canine obesity. *Journal of Small Animal Practice* 2010;51:362–367.
4. Scarlett JM, Donoghue S, Saidla J, Wills J. Overweight cats: Prevalence and risk factors. *International Journal of Obesity and Related Metabolic Disorders* 1994;18:S22–S28.
5. Lund EM, Armstrong PJ, Kirk CA, Klausner JS. Prevalence and risk factors for obesity in adult cats from private US veterinary practices. *International Journal of Applied Research in Veterinary Medicine* 2005;3:88–96.
6. Colliard L, Paragon B-M, Lemuet B, Bénet J-J, Blanchard G. Prevalence and risk factors of obesity in an urban population of healthy cats. *Journal of Feline Medicine and Surgery* 2009;11:35–40.
7. Courcier EA, O'Higgins R, Mellor DJ, Yam PS. Prevalence and risk factors for feline obesity in a first opinion practice in Glasgow, Scotland. *Journal of Feline Medicine and Surgery* 2010;12:746–753.
8. Cave NJ, Allan FJ, Schokkenbroek SL, Metekohy CA, Pfeiffer DU. A cross-sectional study to compare changes in the prevalence and risk factors for feline obesity between 1993 and 2007 in New Zealand Preventative. *Veterinary Medicine* 2012;107:121–133.
9. Rohlf VI, Toukhsati S, Coleman GJ, Bennett PC. Dog obesity: Can dog caregivers' (owners') feeding and exercise intentions and behaviors be predicted from attitudes? *Journal of Applied Animal Welfare Science* 2010;13:213–236.

10. White GA, Hobson-West P, Cobb K, Craigon J, Hammond R, Millar KM. Canine obesity: Is there a difference between veterinarian and owner perception? *Journal of Small Animal Practice* 2011;52:622–626.
11. Bland IM, Guthrie-Jones A, Taylor RD, Hill J. Dog obesity: Owner attitudes and behavior. *Preventative Veterinary Medicine* 2009;92:333–340.
12. Corbee RJ. Obesity in show dogs. *Journal of Animal Physiology and Animal Nutrition* 2013;97:904–910.
13. Corbee RJ. Obesity in show cats. *Journal of Animal Physiology and Animal Nutrition* 2014;98:1075–1080.
14. Murphy M, Lusby AL, Bartges JW, Kirk CA. Size of food bowl and scoop affects amount of food owners feed their dogs. *Journal of Animal Physiology and Animal Nutrition* 2012;96:237–241.
15. German AJ, Holden SL, Mason SL, Bryner C, Bouldoires C, Morris PJ, Deboise M, Biourge V. Imprecision when using measuring cups to weigh out extruded dry kibbled food. *Journal of Animal Physiology and Animal Nutrition* 2011;95:368–373.
16. Linder DE, Freeman LM. Evaluation of calorie density and feeding directions for commercially available diets designed for weight loss in cats and dogs. *Journal of the American Veterinary Medical Association* 2010;236:74–77.
17. Churchill J. Increase the success of weight loss programs by creating an environment for change. *Compendium: Continuing Education for Veterinarians* 2010;32:E1–E4.
18. Linder D, Mueller M. Pet obesity management: Beyond nutrition. *Veterinary Clinics of North America: Small Animal Practice* 2014;44:789–806.
19. Phillips K, Wood F, Kinnersley P. Tackling obesity: The challenge of obesity management for practice nurses in primary care. *Family Practice* 2014;31:51–59.
20. Ogden CL, Carroll MD, Kit BK, Flegal KM. Prevalence of obesity in the United States, 2011–2012. *Journal of the American Medical Association* 2014;311:806–814.
21. Krahn LE, Tovar MD, Miller B. Are pets in the bedroom a problem? *Mayo Clinic Proceedings* 2015;90:1663–1665.
22. German AJ, Holden SL, Wiseman-Orr ML, Reid J, Nolan AM, Biourge V, Morris PJ, Scott EM. Quality of life is reduced in obese dogs but improves after successful weight loss. *Veterinary Journal* 2012;19:428–434.
23. Budge RC, Spicer J, Jones B, St. George R. Health correlates of compatibility and attachment in human-companion animal relationships. *Society and Animals* 1998;6:219–234.
24. Melson GF, Peet S, Sparks C. Children's attachment to their pets: Links to socio-emotional development. *Children's Environments Quarterly* 1992;80:55–65.

25. Kurdek LA. Pet dogs as attachment figures for adult owners. *Journal of Family Psychology* 2009;23:439–446.

26. Stanley IH, Yeates Conwell BA, Bowen C, Van Orden KA. Pet ownership may attenuate loneliness among older adult primary care patients who live alone. *Aging and Mental Health* 2014;18:394–399.

27. Barker SB, Dawson KS. The effects of animal-assisted therapy on anxiety ratings of hospitalized psychiatric patients. *Psychiatric Services* 1998;49:797–801.

28. Kushner RF, Blatner DJ, Jewell DE, Rudloff K. The PPET study: People and pets exercising together. *Obesity (Silver Spring)* 2006;14:1762–1770.

29. Stephens MB, Wilson CC, Goodie JL, Netting FE, Olsen CH, Byers CG. Health perceptions and levels of attachment: Owners and pets exercising together. *Journal of the American Board of Family Medicine* 2012;25:923–926.

7

Role of exercise in the management of obesity

JUSTIN SHMALBERG

7.1 INTRODUCTION

The role of exercise in the management of canine and feline obesity is poorly understood. Inactivity predisposes to the development of canine obesity based on multiple epidemiological studies examining risk factors (1,2). Many veterinarians provide anecdotal recommendations to owners that increasing their overweight or obese pet's exercise will facilitate weight loss. However, the addition of controlled exercise protocols to accepted caloric control measures has not been critically evaluated in the scientific literature. Available evidence in humans suggests that physical activity may have therapeutic benefits during weight loss, but these are often related to cardiovascular health and other secondary changes rather than an effect on caloric intake or the success of a weight loss protocol (3–6). Dogs and cats may derive similar benefits, especially if obese animals have comorbidities such as osteoarthritis, exercise intolerance, and muscle wasting. The impact of exercise on caloric expenditure is related to the distance traveled in normal dogs (7), and if the same is true for overweight animals, there may be a maximum tolerance for exercise in such dogs and cats, which limits the contribution of exercise to energy expenditure.

7.2 EXERCISE AND RISK OF OBESITY

Reduced exercise is a risk factor for canine obesity. One study identified a 4% reduction in the risk of obesity for each hour of weekly exercise (1). A study of Chinese dogs found that dogs permitted free activity were less likely to be obese (OR = 0.685) (8). The magnitude of the difference in activity related to such a reduced risk is often small. For example, obese dogs in Australia exercised on average 2.5 hours per week, whereas nonobese dogs exercised 3.4 hours (2). Dogs that exercised more frequently also did so at a greater speed. Dogs that ran during their exercise were active 50% longer than dogs that walked during exercise. Consequently, those dogs would travel a much greater distance and require greater energy expenditure. Irrespective of the type of exercise performed, each hour was associated with a reduction in obesity risk of 0.9 times (2). Other studies have demonstrated that the steps taken by an animal during a day are inversely related to obesity risk (9). Cats may display similar trends, although the evidence is indirect. Owners of overweight cats potentially interact less with their cats than owners of cats of normal body weight (10). Unfortunately such studies establish only correlations as opposed to causal relationships and should therefore be interpreted with caution. It remains possible that dogs that are obese do not exercise as frequently or as long due to intolerance secondary to increased adiposity or concurrent injuries. For example, there is a correlation between obesity and cranial cruciate ligament rupture (11), which could be a cause of obesity or a sequela that would nonetheless impair activity. Therefore, feeding habits, breed, comorbidities, and owner factors rather than reduced exercise could be the primary causes of obesity (1,11).

Owner habits and attitudes influence an animal's physical activity and could contribute to increased obesity risk, if causality between a reduction in activity and a subsequent increase in body weight were proven. Predictors of the likelihood a dog will exercise include single-dog households, medium and larger dogs, female owners, and households with fewer people (12,13). Owners of obese dogs view exercise less favorably than owners of normal dogs (14), but owner attitudes in a separate study were not correlated to body condition score (15). The available evidence would suggest then that owner's attitude contributes to the amount of exercise a pet receives, but that reduced activity does not definitively cause obesity, as this is likely multifactorial.

7.3 EXERCISE IN THE MANAGEMENT OF HUMAN OBESITY

The link between exercise and obesity management in humans has been more extensively investigated than in dogs or cats. The human literature should be interpreted with caution, however, as a result of species differences. This is true for the dog, which has similar dietary needs to humans, and especially true for the cat, an obligate carnivore. Exercise has been postulated to increase fat oxidation in obese humans, to increase metabolic rate for a period of several hours commensurate with exercise intensity, and to influence the type of secretory cytokine response from muscle, which may counteract some adipokines (16–18). However, dogs display higher basal levels of fat oxidation than humans (7,19,20). The two species demonstrate important differences in adipokine levels during obesity, given that a decrease in total and high molecular weight adiponectin was not observed in dogs following weight loss unlike the observations in human subjects (21). The exercise physiology of cats is poorly described, which further complicates comparisons to the human literature.

The cardiovascular effects of obesity may be mitigated by exercise in humans, whereas the actual effects of activity on measured weight loss are minimal (6). Studies suggest that long-distance exercise (>20 miles weekly) in humans produces body weight losses of less than 0.4% monthly, and that such recommendations are associated with poor compliance (6,22). More modest exercise recommendations appear to reduce the risk of rebound weight gain and to facilitate long-term weight maintenance in people. Such effects were noted at 3 hours of exercise or more weekly, but this is near the baseline activity level documented in some obese dogs (2,6). The monthly rates of weight loss with the addition of exercise to dietary approaches in humans appear greatest at 18 months as compared to those calculated after only 12 months or after 36 months and beyond of follow-up, suggesting that maximal benefit may be significantly delayed and peak at a certain point (23). The heterogeneity of individual responses to exercise and the significant amounts required to achieve a clinical effect are responsible for the clinical recommendation that overweight individuals expect only small amounts of total weight loss from such interventions (<2% starting body weight). However, the combination of moderate-intensity aerobic exercise and diet as opposed to diet alone improves cardiovascular fitness and ameliorates some of the adverse health consequences of obesity such as reduced cardiac function, increased blood pressure, insulin resistance and diabetes mellitus, and dyslipidemia (3–5). Such benefits may be realized in dogs and cats, but species differences influence the applicability of these findings, and further research is required. For example, obesity in cats and humans, but not in dogs, is associated with non-insulin-dependent diabetes mellitus. However, the role of exercise in reducing diabetic morbidity and mortality in cats has not been explored.

7.4 COMORBIDITIES, EXERCISE, AND OBESITY IN DOGS AND IN CATS

A number of comorbidities are associated with canine or feline obesity, which are described in detail elsewhere (Chapter 3), and are potentially relevant to exercise protocols recommended for obese patients. Limited data suggest that obesity affects cardiovascular fitness in dogs as in humans. A reduction in exercise tolerance as well as a notable increase in left atrial pressure and mild increase in blood pressure have been documented in dogs (24). Airway resistance is altered in some obese dogs during hyperpnea, which could be one factor in the anecdotally observed resistance of some overweight animals to exercise (25). Increasing adiposity predisposes to radiographic and clinical signs of canine osteoarthritis (26), but interestingly, experimental models of repetitive exercise in which dogs were fitted with additive weights and run on treadmills failed to document an increased severity of arthritis as compared to control animals (27). This may suggest that the hormonal impacts of obesity cause arthritis, or that in animals genetically predisposed to arthritis, increased articular loading worsens the condition only after it develops. Alternatively, obesity may reduce activity, which could be associated with a decline in the mechanical forces that contribute to the health and nutrition of chondrocytes (28). Regular low-impact exercise has been recommended for the management of arthritis in humans and in dogs (29,30), and weight reduction improved weight-bearing in osteoarthritic animals and reduced markers of systemic inflammation (21,31). The performance and efficacy of various exercise protocols in cats has not received significant attention from the scientific literature.

7.5 USE OF EXERCISE IN CANINE AND FELINE OBESITY PROTOCOLS

Exercise is thought to contribute to the efficacy of a weight loss program, but this is based primarily on expert opinion and not on clinical trials (32). Recommendations are not derived from peer-reviewed prospective investigations, but commonly suggest that pets walk for 30 minutes or less, or that they swim for 15 minutes daily, five to seven times weekly (10). Consensus weight management recommendations also recommend enrichment activities for cats and walking for overweight dogs but without detailed or evidence-based suggestions (33). Few studies are available to determine the best role, if any, of exercise in canine and feline weight loss protocols.

Overweight dogs with greater pedometer-reported physical activity were able to consume more energy (54 kcal per metabolic body weight [MBW]) than were inactive dogs (42 kcal per MBW) (34). Each 1000-step interval showed a mild correlation to a 1 kcal/kg$^{0.75}$ increase in energy intake (r = 0.36). An underwater treadmill was incorporated into a program that achieved 1.5% of weight loss weekly in overweight dogs (35). Dogs being calorically restricted with a therapeutic weight loss diet also received an average of 13 hydrotherapy sessions and walked an average distance of 0.97 km. Owners were also asked to walk dogs daily, but this was not quantified. The authors suggest that the rate of weight loss was greater than historical controls, but unfortunately multiple interventions were retrospectively evaluated in the analysis. Osteoarthritic overweight dogs subjected to an at-home and in-clinic physiotherapy program lost 46% more weight than did control animals receiving caloric restriction and instructions for owner-driven physical therapy alone (36). Physiotherapy primarily involved active exercises at home starting at 1 hour of walking, but, unfortunately, the caloric intake of the two groups was not provided.

The most representative data of veterinary-led exercise interventions is derived from a recent study of a weight loss program with incorporated dietary management alone or diet plus thrice weekly hydrotherapy (30 minutes) and land-based treadmill walking (30 minutes) in a small group of overweight dogs (37). Inclines, walking or trotting speeds, and water depth were adjusted to the treated patients, and owners were encouraged to exercise treated dogs at home, whereas owners of diet-only dogs were not given such advice. Energy intake was not different between groups during the study. Mean weight loss in exercised dogs was 1.16% weekly for 12 weeks, and 1.08% weekly for dietary management exclusively, which was not statistically significant. An improvement in resting heart rate was observed in both groups but was not different between groups, despite increased accelerometry counts in treated dogs and decreased counts in diet-only dogs. The primary significant finding, and possible benefit to exercise therapy, was an increase in lean body mass with exercise (+4.6%) versus a decrease in sedentary dogs (−2.5%).

Possibly advantageous changes in the relevant transcriptome were identified in enrolled dogs in a related study (38). The difference in weight loss, if statistically relevant, would amount to 330 grams over the study period; applying Wishnofsky's rule (39), this would be an endogenous energy consumption of 2500 kcal, or about 182 $kcal/kg^{0.75}$, as a result of 36 hours of exercise covering an estimated distance of 19.7 km. The resulting value suggests, if ascribed solely to the treadmill exercise performed in the clinic, a distance-based energy cost of 9.2 $kcal/kg^{0.75}/km$. Treated dogs displayed an increase in weekly accelerometry counts of 0.85 million weekly compared to baseline, for an energy per count value of 245 kcal per million counts. Interestingly, diet-only dogs had a 7.6% decrease at 12 weeks in accelerometry counts as compared to baseline, which is roughly consistent with another study of diet only that documented an 11.3% decrease at the same time point (40).

The energy expenditure of various types of activity is known for normal, fit dogs (Figure 7.1) (7,41,42). Sitting and standing require 30% and 46% more energy, respectively, than lying down, and therefore sustained modest changes in a dog's activity could influence daily calorie expenditure (43). Walking dogs require about 1.2 $kcal/kg^{0.75}/km$, and therefore a medium-sized dog may only increase its energy expenditure by 1% over the course of 30 minutes of walking as commonly suggested (44). The energy required for running dogs is approximately 1.1 kcal/kg/km; dogs with longer legs use less energy to cover a fixed distance as compared to those with shorter legs (7,45), but most obese dogs are too poorly conditioned to run. Underwater treadmill activity in elbow-height water requires 1.9 $kcal/kg^{0.75}/km$ (44). A 30-minute session of underwater treadmill administered to a medium-sized dog would increase daily energy expenditure by only 1.5% (42). No data are available on which to evaluate the recommendation that animals swim to improve weight loss success.

An enrichment program in cats which employed effort-driven feeding dispensers, new toys and climbing structures, and food-incentivized exercises, produced an unquantified increase in activity when paired with a therapeutic diet, resulting in a statistically significant, but clinically insignificant, reduction in body weight as compared to controls (46). Extension of the photoperiod provided to cats to 16 hours of light per day increased activity counts by 20%, but only increased energy intake 5% (47). Conflicting studies are available on whether increased feeding frequency or dietary moisture increases activity in cats (48,49).

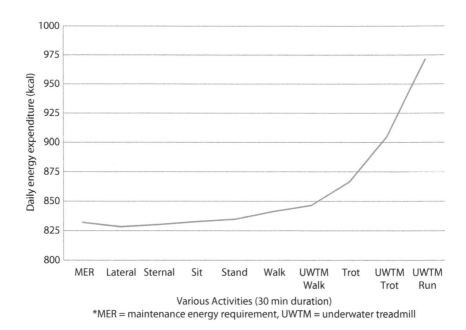

Figure 7.1 Comparative increases in caloric expenditure with various exercises performed for 30 minutes by a 20 kg healthy dog in normal body condition.

All exercise recommendations are provided to an owner and are consequently dependent on owner compliance. The same factors that impair exercise before initiation of a weight loss protocol are likely to remain unless the owner strongly commits to this part of the weight loss plan. Pedometer data from an obesity clinic demonstrates that in spite of a recommendation to exercise obese dogs, the average recorded daily steps remained the same throughout a 10-week program (9). The authors suggest that this is due to owner behavior, but it could also be due to physical limits, intolerance, or learned behavior. A separate study also failed to document an increase in activity after weight loss, which may suggest that a reduction in adiposity does not change owner or dog behavior (40). Owners frequently and subjectively report that their pet is "active" and receiving routine exercise, but this has rarely been corroborated in scientific study (10). No studies have yet assessed ways to improve adherence to exercise recommendations in overweight pets. However, one study of a combined human and pet weight loss and exercise program documented that dogs lost weight concurrently with their owners (50). Interestingly, the rate of weight loss of the owners who exercised with their pet was not different than those who exercised alone.

7.6 PRACTICAL RECOMMENDATIONS

- Increased exercise in the absence of caloric restriction is unlikely to result in clinically significant weight loss.

- Exercise appears to preserve lean body mass during caloric restriction.
- Physical activity likely exerts greater benefits on overall systemic health than on the rate of weight loss, and any activity should consider comorbidities or desired health effects, such as osteoarthritis, cardiovascular fitness, or exercise tolerance.
- The distance, rather than the duration, of exercise should be the emphasis of any recommendations because the distance traveled is the primary determinant of energy expenditure in normal, and presumably obese, dogs.
- Most owners will be unable to walk their dogs for a sufficient distance to achieve significant increases in energy expenditure; an hour of walking produces only a small increase in daily energy expenditure.
- Underwater treadmill walking results in increased energy expenditure over a fixed distance as compared to walking, but for the benefits to be realized, the frequency must be equal or greater to that which the owner can provide with conventional walking.
- The alteration of feeding frequency may increase activity level in cats, and there is no disadvantage to feeding an increased number of meals if the owner's schedule permits.
- Owner education about exercise is critical, and recommendations must be considered in the context of the owner's lifestyle and personal beliefs.

7.7 CONCLUSION

Exercise in the absence of significant caloric restriction is unlikely to result in significant weight loss. The role of exercise in the management of obesity should therefore focus on the benefits of exercise for other purposes, such as increasing endurance, improving the rehabilitation or management of comorbidities, or enhancing cardiovascular fitness. The use of veterinary-assisted exercise modalities for weight loss, such as underwater treadmill therapy, may not produce sufficient additive benefits to justify the expense and effort unless done on a routine basis. Methods of increasing feline activity are poorly described, as are the therapeutic implications of exercise on obesity in cats. Additional studies are required on the energy consumption of obese animals during different activities as are prospective controlled trials of such interventions.

REFERENCES

1. Courcier EA, Thomson RM, Mellor DJ, Yam PS. An epidemiological study of environmental factors associated with canine obesity. *Journal of Small Animal Practice* 2010;51(7):362–367.
2. Robertson ID. The association of exercise, diet and other factors with owner-perceived obesity in privately owned dogs from metropolitan Perth, WA. *Preventive Veterinary Medicine* 2003;58(1):75–83.
3. De Feo P. Is high-intensity exercise better than moderate-intensity exercise for weight loss? *Nutrition, Metabolism and Cardiovascular Diseases* 2013;23(11):1037–1042.

4. Lee DC, Sui X, Blair SN. Does physical activity ameliorate the health hazards of obesity? *British Journal of Sports Medicine* 2009;43(1):49–51.
5. Swift DL, Johannsen NM, Lavie CJ, Earnest CP, Church TS. The role of exercise and physical activity in weight loss and maintenance. *Progress in Cardiovascular Diseases* 2014;56(4):441–447.
6. Wadden TA, Webb VL, Moran CH, Bailer BA. Lifestyle modification for obesity: New developments in diet, physical activity, and behavior therapy. *Circulation* 2012;125(9):1157–1170.
7. National Research Council Ad Hoc Committee on Dog and Cat Nutrition. *Nutrient Requirements of Dogs and Cats.* Washington DC: National Academies Press; 2006.
8. Mao J, Xia Z, Chen J, Yu J. Prevalence and risk factors for canine obesity surveyed in veterinary practices in Beijing, China. *Preventive Veterinary Medicine* 2013;112(3):438–442.
9. Warren BS, Wakshlag JJ, Maley M, Farrell TJ, Struble AM, Panasevich MR, Wells MT. Use of pedometers to measure the relationship of dog walking to body condition score in obese and non-obese dogs. *British Journal of Nutrition* 2011;106(S1):S85–S89.
10. Roudebush P, Schoenherr WD, Delaney SJ. An evidence-based review of the use of therapeutic foods, owner education, exercise, and drugs for the management of obese and overweight pets. *Journal of the American Veterinary Medical Association* 2008;233(5):717–725.
11. Lund EM, Armstrong PJ, Kirk CA, Klausner JS. Prevalence and risk factors for obesity in adult dogs from private US veterinary practices. *International Journal of Applied Research in Veterinary Medicine* 2006;4(2):177.
12. Degeling C, Burton L, McCormack GR. An investigation of the association between socio-demographic factors, dog-exercise requirements, and the amount of walking dogs receive. *Canadian Journal of Veterinary Research* 2012;76(3):235.
13. Westgarth C, Christian HE, Christley RM. Factors associated with daily walking of dogs. *BMC Veterinary Research* 2015;11:116. doi:10.1186/s12917-015-0434-5.
14. Kienzle E, Bergler R, Mandernach A. A comparison of the feeding behavior and the human-animal relationship in owners of normal and obese dogs. *Journal of Nutrition* 1998;128(12 Suppl): 2779S–2782S.
15. Rohlf VI, Toukhsati S, Coleman GJ, Bennett PC. Dog obesity: Can dog caregivers' (owners') feeding and exercise intentions and behaviors be predicted from attitudes? *Journal of Applied Animal Welfare Science* 2010;13(3):213–236.
16. Blaak EE, Wim HMS. Substrate oxidation, obesity and exercise training. *Best Practice & Research Clinical Endocrinology & Metabolism* 2002;16(4):667–678.
17. Borsheim E, Bahr R. Effect of exercise intensity, duration and mode on post-exercise oxygen consumption. *Sports Medicine* 2003;33(14):1037–1060.

18. Pedersen BK, Febbraio MA. Muscles, exercise and obesity: Skeletal muscle as a secretory organ. *Nature Reviews Endocrinology* 2012;8(8):457–465.

19. Havel RJ, Naimark A, Borchgrevink CF. Turnover rate and oxidation of free fatty acids of blood plasma in man during exercise: Studies during continuous infusion of palmitate-1–C14. *Journal of Clinical Investigation* 1963;42(7):1054.

20. Issekutz B, Miller HI, Paul P, Rodahl K. Source of fat oxidation in exercising dogs. *American Journal of Physiology* 1964;207(3):583–589.

21. Wakshlag JJ, Struble AM, Levine CB, Bushey JJ, Laflamme DP, Long GM. The effects of weight loss on adipokines and markers of inflammation in dogs. *British Journal of Nutrition* 2011;106(Suppl 1):S11–S14. doi:10.1017/S0007114511000560.

22. Slentz CA, Duscha BD, Johnson JL, Ketchum K, Aiken LB, Samsa GP, Houmard JA, Bales CW, Kraus WE. Effects of the amount of exercise on body weight, body composition, and measures of central obesity: STRRIDE—A randomized controlled study. *Archives of Internal Medicine* 2004;164(1):31–39.

23. Avenell A, Brown TJ, McGee MA, Campbell MK, Grant AM, Broom J, Jung RT, Smith WCS. What interventions should we add to weight reducing diets in adults with obesity? A systematic review of randomized controlled trials of adding drug therapy, exercise, behaviour therapy or combinations of these interventions. *Journal of Human Nutrition and Dietetics* 2004;17(4):293–316.

24. Leland MH, Edwards TC, Montant J-P. Abnormal cardiovascular responses to exercise during the development of obesity in dogs. *American Journal of Hypertension* 1994;7(4 Pt 1):374–378.

25. Bach JF, Rozanski EA, Bedenice D, Chan DL, Freeman LM, Lofgren JL, Oura TJ, Hoffman AM. Association of expiratory airway dysfunction with marked obesity in healthy adult dogs. *American Journal of Veterinary Research* 2007;68(6):670–675. doi:10.2460/ajvr.68.6.670.

26. Smith GK, Lawler DF, Biery DN, Powers MY, Shofer F, Gregor TP, Karbe GT, McDonald-Lynch MB, Evans RH, Kealy RD. Chronology of hip dysplasia development in a cohort of 48 Labrador retrievers followed for life. *Veterinary Surgery* 2012;41(1):20–33. doi:10.1111/j.1532–950X.2011.00935.x.

27. Newton PM, Mow VC, Gardner TR, Buckwalter JA, Albright JP. The effect of lifelong exercise on canine articular cartilage. *The American Journal of Sports Medicine* 1997;25(3):282–287.

28. Griffin TM, Guilak F. The role of mechanical loading in the onset and progression of osteoarthritis. *Exercise and Sports Sciences Reviews* 2005;33(4):195–200.

29. Bennell KL, Hinman RS. A review of the clinical evidence for exercise in osteoarthritis of the hip and knee. *Journal of Science and Medicine in Sport* 2011;14(1):4–9. doi:10.1016/j.jsams.2010.08.002.

30. Johnston SA, McLaughlin RM, Budsberg SC. Nonsurgical management of osteoarthritis in dogs. *Veterinary Clinics of North America: Small Animal Practice* 2008;38(6):1449–1470.
31. Impellizeri JA, Tetrick MA, Muir P. Effect of weight reduction on clinical signs of lameness in dogs with hip osteoarthritis. *Journal of the American Veterinary Medical Association* 2000;216(7):1089–1091.
32. Linder D, Mueller M. Pet obesity management: Beyond nutrition. *Veterinary Clinics of North America: Small Animal Practice* 2014;44(4):789–806.
33. Brooks D, Churchill J, Fein K, Linder D, Michel KE, Tudor K, Ward E, Witzel A. 2014 AAHA weight management guidelines for dogs and cats. *Journal of the American Animal Hospital Association* 2014;50(1):1–11.
34. Wakshlag JJ, Struble AM, Warren BS, Maley M, Panasevich MR, Cummings KJ, Long GM, Laflamme DE. Evaluation of dietary energy intake and physical activity in dogs undergoing a controlled weight-loss program. *Journal of the American Veterinary Medical Association* 2012;240(4):413–419. doi:10.2460/javma.240.4.413.
35. Chauvet A, Laclair J, Elliott DA, German AJ. Incorporation of exercise, using an underwater treadmill, and active client education into a weight management program for obese dogs. *The Canadian Veterinary Journal* 2011;52(5):491–496.
36. Mlacnik E, Bockstahler BA, Müller M, Tetrick MA, Nap RC, Zentek J. Effects of caloric restriction and a moderate or intense physiotherapy program for treatment of lameness in overweight dogs with osteoarthritis. *Journal of the American Veterinary Medical Association* 2006;229(11):1756–1760. doi:10.2460/javma.229.11.1756.
37. Vitger AD, Stallknecht BM, Nielsen DH, Bjornvad CR. Integration of a physical training program in a weight loss plan for overweight pet dogs. *Journal of American Veterinary Medical Association* 2016;248(2):174–182.
38. Uribe JH, Vitger AD, Ritz C, Fredholm M, Bjornvad CR, Cirera S. Physical training and weight loss in dogs lead to transcriptional changes in genes involved in the glucose transport pathway in muscle and adipose tissues. *The Veterinary Journal* 2016;208:22–27.
39. Thomas DM, Gonzalez MC, Pereira AZ, Redman LM, and Heymsfield SB, Time to correctly predict the amount of weight loss with dieting. *Journal of the Academy of Nutrition and Dietetics* 2014;114(6): 857–861.
40. Morrison R, Reilly JJ, Penpraze V, Pendlebury E, Yam PS. A 6–month observational study of changes in objectively measured physical activity during weight loss in dogs. *Journal of Small Animal Practice* 2014;55(11):566–570.
41. Shmalberg J. Part 1: Canine performance nutrition. *Today's Veterinary Practice* 2014;4(6):72–76.
42. Shmalberg J. Part 2: Canine rehabilitative nutrition. *Today's Veterinary Practice* 2014;5(1):87–90.

43. Scott KC, Shmalberg J, Williams JM, Morris PJ, Hill RC. Energy intake of pet dogs compared to energy expenditure at rest, sitting, and standing. *The WALTHAM International Nutritional Sciences Symposium 2013*. Portland, Oregon; 2013.

44. Shmalberg J, Scott KC, Williams JM, Hill RC. Energy expenditure of dogs exercising on an underwater treadmill compared to that on a dry treadmill. *13th Annual AAVN Clinical Nutrition and Research Symposium*. Seattle, Washington; 2013.

45. Hill RC, Scott KC, Williams JM, Morris PJ, Shmalberg J. Energy required for trotting is inversely proportional to leg length in small dogs. *13th Annual AAVN Clinical Nutrition and Research Symposium*, Seattle, Washington; 2013.

46. Clarke DL, Wrigglesworth D, Holmes K, Hackett R, Michel K. Using environmental and feeding enrichment to facilitate feline weight loss. *Journal of Animal Physiology and Animal Nutrition* 2005;89(11–12):427.

47. Kappen KL, Garner LM, Kerr KR, Swanson KS. Effects of photoperiod on food intake, activity and metabolic rate in adult neutered male cats. *Journal of Animal Physiology and Animal Nutrition* 2014;98(5):958–967.

48. de Godoy MRC, Ochi K, de Oliveira Mateus LF, de Justino ACC, Swanson KS. Feeding frequency, but not dietary water content, affects voluntary physical activity in young lean adult female cats. *Journal of Animal Science* 2015;93(5):2597–2601.

49. Deng P, Iwazaki E, Suchy SA, Pallotto MR, Swanson KS. Effects of feeding frequency and dietary water content on voluntary physical activity in healthy adult cats. *Journal of Animal Science* 2014;92(3):1271–1277.

50. Kushner RF, Blatner DJ, Jewell DE, Rudloff K. The PPET study: People and pets exercising together. *Obesity (Silver Spring)* 2006;14(10):1762–1770. doi:10.1038/oby.2006.203.

8

Establishing a weight management program in clinical practice

MARYANNE MURPHY, ALEXANDER J. GERMAN,
AND MARTHA G. CLINE

8.1 INTRODUCTION

Veterinarians and veterinary nurses in general or community practice are encouraged to create comprehensive programs to provide clients with weight loss services for their pets. Consultation for weight loss not only includes the initial examination and feeding program development, but also months of follow-up during both the weight loss and weight maintenance phases. Support after weight loss for these pets is vital to help them maintain a healthy body condition and avoid the pitfalls of potential weight regain. Here, the owner must be taught to change their relationship with their pet permanently, so as to maintain control of food intake and activity levels (1,2). Several steps can be taken to improve success with the initial weight loss consultation as well as the long-term follow-up to improve long-term outcomes (3–6).

8.2 INITIAL CONSULTATION

8.2.1 Diet, activity, and household history

Before the first appointment for weight management, the owner should be asked to complete a diet, activity, and household history form (DAHHF; Appendix 8.1). Ideally, the owner is given instructions to complete the form in an Internet-based submission format or a paper copy that is posted to them when scheduling the consultation. Submission of the form in advance of the appointment ensures the veterinary team has time to properly review the information prior to the appointment. If not completed in advance, the DAHHF may be filled out in the office, but this is less desirable since, as has been documented in people, owners may not recall precise names of diets, treats or supplements, or actual quantities fed to their pets (7,8). The time needed to properly fill out the DAHHF will also likely cause a delay in the hospital schedule unless either built into the appointment slot or unless the owner is instructed to arrive at least 10–15 minutes early.

The DAHHF should be utilized to obtain the caloric content of diets, treats (commercial and table foods), and food used for medication administration to calculate total current daily caloric intake prior to the appointment. The written information should be checked and verified during the appointment, with further questioning used to prompt or remind the owner about food items they might have forgotten. It helps to have more than one family member present during review of the diet history to account for all food items. Many owners may also not be aware that supplements often contain calories (e.g., fish oil, soft chews) and these should also be counted toward daily intake.

In addition to knowledge of the dietary history, the DAHHF also prompts the owner for critical information about the family unit (including all family members and pets) and also the activity that the animal undertakes. For the family unit, information should be gathered regarding details on each family member (age and sex) and who is responsible for feeding, treating, and exercising the animal. It is also necessary to know about other pets (age, sex, breed, neuter status, etc.) and their relationship with the animal being enrolled (i.e., are they related, are they fed together, are they exercised together, or do they get along).

A veterinary nurse or assistant may be assigned to complete this task to improve appointment efficiency, but they should be experienced in taking such a history. If a DAHHF is not completed at any point prior to the appointment, asking owners to supply more detailed information following the initial consultation may be helpful. A reminder phone call or e-mail is recommended within 24 hours of the consultation if the owner does not provide the DAHHF within this time period.

8.2.2 Resources used during initial consultation

Once the background information has been gathered, including the nutritional assessment (see Chapter 5), the current weight and body condition score (BCS) should be illustrated for the owner against their pet's expected ideal weight goals (see Chapter 5). Various systems for scoring body condition are available, with five, seven, or nine categories (9–12). However, recently, the World Small Animal Veterinary Association (WSAVA) Global Nutrition Committee has recommended universal adoption of the 9-point BCS in both dogs and cats, and non-branded BCS forms (see Chapter 5) are available on its website and can be given to owners to illustrate their pet's current BCS against expected final goals (13,14).

Photographs of the pet from multiple angles while standing (i.e., dorsal, lateral; Figure 8.1) are recommended at the initial consultation as well. These should be used to compare to final pictures once the pet has reached target body weight (see Chapter 5) (15). These photographs may be used for a variety of purposes such as creating a weight loss success board to display in the clinic, marketing, or education. Owners should sign a release form at the initial appointment if photographs are to be used for marketing or displayed to the public. An example photo release form is provided in Appendix 8.2.

Many owners will want to provide treats during their pet's weight loss program. It is worth having prepared lists of calorie information for commonly used human foods, commercial treats, or potentially a homemade treat recipe that can be provided to the owners either in person or e-mailed after the appointment. Owners may also use a daily treat allowance sheet (Appendix 8.3) at home each day to clearly illustrate how they are utilizing their treat allowances and to avoid providing excess treat calories. Treat allowances and individual treat recommendations should be tailored to be appropriate when comorbidities requiring nutritional intervention are present (e.g., fat or protein restriction). It is also useful to provide the owners with a weekly food diary (Appendix 8.4), where they record food offered, food consumed, activity, "confessions" (e.g., occasions when additional food has been consumed, be it stolen by the animal or given by the owner as a treat), activity, demeanor, and any other observations (such as other illnesses).

At the conclusion of the appointment, the owners should be given a range of tools to assist them with the weight loss process, in the form of a weight loss starter kit. If possible, free samples or specific product recommendations should be given. Suggested items include:

- Sample of canned or dry food
- Leashes (consider hospital branded)
- Gram scales, or appropriately sized measuring cups (e.g., 1 cup, 1/3 cup, 1/4 cup, 1/8 cup), if the owner will not accept the use of gram scales for measuring food

(a)

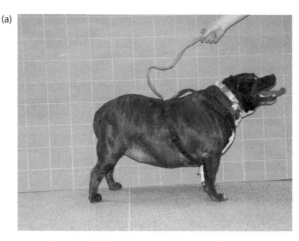

(b)

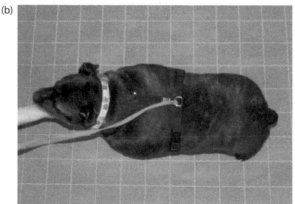

Figure 8.1 Photographs taken during initial consultation. These should be used to compare to final pictures once the pet has reached target body weight. (Photographs courtesy of the University of Liverpool Royal Canin Weight Management Clinic.)

- Treats with caloric content clearly defined, and instructions on how much to feed
- Toys and puzzle feeders
- Other relevant items that might be available including waste bags, food bowls, etc.

Not uncommonly, the manufacturers of various therapeutic weight loss products will be happy to supply samples of their products for this purpose.

In addition to the aforementioned resources, further support should be considered in the form of organized group meetings, whereby owners can meet to share their experiences. During these sessions, veterinary staff conveying simple tips for weight management can give short educational talks. Owners of dogs should be encouraged to bring their dog, provided that there are no behavioral concerns; however, cat sessions are better conducted without the pets present. Such sessions may provide camaraderie among owners struggling with the same problems, such as dealing with begging behavior or food seeking and tips on increasing play activity. If possible, it is helpful to have owners whose dogs have already completed the weight loss phase (and are now maintaining weight) in addition to those on the weight loss program. This enables sharing of good practice among clients and also reinforces the need for owners to continue with programs even after the weight loss phase has ended.

If face-to-face meetings are not possible or there is insufficient interest from owners, an alternative would be to consider the use of running an online forum or listserv, which is moderated by a member of the weight management team. These can be very successful but do take time to administer, which should be considered from a staffing and cost point of view. Finally, the practice could facilitate opportunities for clients to interact among one another, for example, via a walking group for committed dog owners. These can be easy to establish since the impetus to establish and maintain them comes from the owner rather than the practice.

8.2.3 Quick tips

- Completion of a DAHHF by the owner at home, rather than in the office, to obtain a more accurate history prior to the initial consultation is recommended.
- Use an assigned veterinary nurse or assistant to research calorie contents of diet and treats to calculate total current caloric intake.
- Provide the owner with an illustrated sheet to demonstrate current body condition against expected final goals.
- Take pictures of the patient at the initial consultation to be compared to pictures once the patient has reached their ideal body weight.
- Have owners sign a photo release form.
- Provide owners with daily treat allowance sheets and weekly food diaries.
- Provide a weight loss kit, including samples of the recommended diet(s), at the conclusion of the consultation.
- Consider establishing a support group for owners to provide encouragement and share weight loss success stories.

8.3 FOLLOW-UP AND RECHECK APPOINTMENTS

It is good practice to contact the owner, by phone or e-mail, 24 hours after their first appointment to ensure that they are happy and have not had any immediate concerns. There can be a lot for an owner to consider at this first appointment, and it is not uncommon for confusion to arise or for there to be some problems with implementing the new regime. Not only do owners value this contact, but it can help to maintain compliance, making them less likely to subsequently drop out (16).

Recheck appointments should then be organized on a regular schedule, every 2–4 weeks, depending upon clinic routine, owner availability, and progress with the program. Ideally, all owners should be encouraged to return every 2 weeks initially, since this can be a time when frequent counseling and alterations are needed. If the initial food allocation is correct, all obese animals should lose at least some weight at this stage. This initial recheck is a way of confirming the success of the program with the owner and reassuring them it has been worthwhile. For pets reliably losing weight, in-clinic weight rechecks may be alternated with at-home weight sessions in which the owner weighs their pet on a home scale and contacts the clinic with scheduled weight updates. In the authors' experience, this method is more likely to be associated with poor long-term adherence to the weight loss program and should be used sparingly and only with pets in later stages of their weight loss program. Additionally, weighing large dogs on a home scale intended for people may be cumbersome. In-clinic weight checks on a regular basis using the same scale remain the preferred method to ensure consistent weight loss success. Owners should also be provided with free access to a clinic scale to check the weight of their pet at any time during office hours.

Weight recheck appointments should be scheduled prior to the owner leaving the building. Prescheduling appointments greatly improves long-term follow-up and compliance (16). All appointments should ideally be confirmed 24 hours in advance and may be arranged for a shorter time period than that used for other appointments. Consider recording these as veterinary nurse appointments. Clinic nurses should be trained to review total calorie intake, determine current weight and BCS, and calculate rate of weight loss. If weight loss is outside the recommended range (see Chapter 5), lack of owner compliance is suspected, or the patient has reached their ideal body weight and condition, follow-up with the veterinarian is recommended.

There are many approaches to monitoring progress via body weight, BCS, body shape (using a tape measure), and photography. Body weight measurements alone can be used to determine the efficacy of a weight loss program and should be the principle outcome measure used for decision making (17). In contrast, changes in BCS occur slowly (typically requiring 5%–15% body weight loss per BCS unit on a 9-point scale) (18) and are better assessed periodically rather than at every visit. Tape measure assessments can be imprecise (19), not least if undertaken by different people, and are best used to complement other measures to demonstrate change.

For most obese dogs and cats, the weight loss phase is likely to last at least 6 months, with the duration of some lasting beyond a year (20). The vast majority will require alterations to the program during this time if progress stalls (e.g., lack of weight loss or gain in weight between checks). Usually, it is necessary to reduce food allocation, usually by a small amount (e.g., a maximum of 5%–10% of the allocation). If dry food and gram scales are used, these small implements can be delivered with great accuracy; it can be more challenging to make accurate adjustments when using wet food or measuring food with a cup (21,22). In cases where weight loss progresses too quickly (e.g., >3%/week for more than two visits), a small increase in food intake can be considered; however, in the authors' experience, such occasions are rare. Progress with weight loss is usually good in the first 3–6 months, but inevitably becomes more challenging thereafter. Later on, slower rates of weight loss are acceptable (e.g., ∼0.3%–0.5%/week) provided that the owner remains motivated and is happy to stick to the program (see Box 8.1 for incentive ideas).

8.3.1 Quick tips

- Contact owners within 24 hours of the initial consultation to address any immediate concern.
- Provide owners with free-of-charge access to a clinic scale to weigh their pets at any time during office hours.
- Recommend weight recheck appointments every 2–4 weeks, initially, with longer intervals subsequently being allowed between checks if progress is good.
- Recheck appointments should be booked prior to the owner leaving the building and ideally confirmed 24 hours in advance.
- Veterinary nurses can perform weight rechecks once they have had appropriate training.
- Adjust food intake throughout the weight loss phase and encourage use of gram scales to improve accuracy and precision of amounts being offered.

BOX 8.1: Special focus on incentives

The weight loss and target weight maintenance process is immensely challenging for the owner, and it is not uncommon for their resolve to weaken, increasing the chance that the process will stall. Therefore, it is helpful to implement a system of rewards and affirmations for clients and their pets who reach key milestones in order to improve owner adherence to the weight loss and maintenance recommendations (1,2). The exact points for awarding rewards can be determined by the individual practice, based upon resources available. The following four milestones are suggested:

1. *6% body weight loss.* Evidence suggests that there are measurable improvements in health by this point in the weight loss program (3). A simple reward, such as a rosette or certificate would be suitable. However, since animals will be more mobile at this point, a toy reward could be considered.
2. *Half-way to target (e.g., 10% starting weight loss if a total 20% weight loss is required).* An excellent milestone since being closer to the end than the beginning can provide motivation to stick with the plan. Owners may be experiencing decreased resolve to ignore begging activity at this stage (4), so a puzzle feeder or similar stimulus might be a suitable reward.
3. *Three-quarter distance.* By this stage, weight loss may be slow and increasingly challenging. An incentive at this point can help to motivate clients in the final stages. Since owners who make it this far are likely to be motivated to continue, providing some of the food free of charge could be a valued incentive for all their hard work to date. Therapeutic

weight loss diet manufacturers may be willing to provide samples for these patients.

4. *Achievement of target weight.* Similar items can be considered to those already discussed.

REFERENCES

1. Webb TL. Why pet owners overfeed: A self-regulation perspective. In: *Companion Animal Nutrition Summit: The Future of Weight Management.* Barcelona, Spain: Nestle Purina; 2015, pp. 89–94.
2. Murphy M. Obesity treatment: Environment and behavior modification. *The Veterinary Clinics of North America: Small Animal Practice* 2016;46:883–898.
3. Marshall WG, Hazewinkel HAW, Mullen D et al. The effect of weight loss on lameness in obese dogs with osteoarthritis. *Veterinary Research Communications* 2010;34:241–253.
4. Bissot T, Servet E, Vidal S et al. Novel dietary strategies can improve the outcome of weight loss programmes in obese client-owned cats. *Journal of Feline Medicine and Surgery* 2010;12:104–112.

8.4 MAINTENANCE APPOINTMENTS

Once the patient has reached ideal body weight and condition, resources to acknowledge success should be provided. Photographs of the patient can be taken to compare to the "before" photos. Consider providing the owner with a certificate detailing starting weight, BCS, body fat percentage (estimated vs. quantified using morphometric measurements) compared to final check in values. Also consider providing the pet with branded items to indicate successful weight loss at the clinic such as a bandanna, collar, or leash. Weight loss success boards displayed within the hospital are an excellent way to demonstrate to other owners the success of the program and encourage them to sign up. Highlight successful weight loss patients (e.g., hospital "star slimmers") on a monthly or quarterly basis, based on an animal and owner pair who has made particularly good progress with their program. The criteria for selection of winners can be kept flexible, so as to enable the award to be given for various reasons. That way, if needed, it can be used in a timely fashion for a particular client to help motivate them when required.

At the time of completion of the weight loss phase, it is also sensible to have an information pack available that prepares the client for the maintenance phase. This packet should include updated feeding recommendations to help the pet successfully maintain its newly achieved healthier body condition. It is common for owners (and indeed veterinary professionals) to believe that the process has been completed and to allow bad habits to recur, which were likely associated with the original weight gain. Studies have indicated that approximately half of all dogs and cats that successfully reach their target weight regain some weight at this point (5,6). Therefore, time should be taken to implement a program of follow-up for the weight management process. Initially, maintenance rechecks should return to occurring every 2–4 weeks, while the food intake is gradually increased in small increments (a maximum of 5%–10% at a time). Once the target weight has been maintained over at least two consecutive appointments, the interval between checks can be extended gradually (e.g., to every 4–8 weeks, then every 3 months, and a minimum of every 6 months thereafter). Consider utilizing a discounted rate for these appointments, especially if performed by a veterinary nurse. However, if weight gain and noncompliance are encountered, follow-up with the veterinarian is recommended to create new weight loss recommendations.

There can be many reasons for why a particular animal will regain weight after successfully reaching their target body weight, but a key factor is the type of food used during the maintenance period. Indeed, animals that remain on the same food that was used for weight loss (e.g., a purpose-formulated weight management food) are 20 times less likely to regain weight during follow-up, albeit fed at an increased amount so as to maintain weight (5). Given the added cost of such foods, owners may be reluctant to continue with feeding the food long-term. If feasible, it might be worth offering the food at a discounted rate so as to ensure their compliance.

8.4.1 Quick tips

- Provide the owner with a certificate, before and after photographs, and/or hospital-branded gifts to acknowledge the pet's weight loss success.
- Consider a weight loss success board to display in the clinic lobby.
- Create a maintenance phase packet to prepare the owner for the road ahead.
- Devote as much attention to the weight maintenance period as to weight loss, so as to ensure rebound is spotted early and rectified.
- Recommend weight rechecks more frequently initially, with progression to a maximum of every 6 months to maintain accountability.
- Recommend that owners continue to feed the purpose-formulated weight management diet during the maintenance period, and offer it to them at a discount.

8.5 GETTING THE WORD OUT

When implementing weight management services within a practice, it is recommended to prepare succinct marketing materials in the form of a handout, pamphlet, or informational page on the hospital's website. Information should include reasoning behind the program, structure (i.e., initial consult followed by a set number of weight rechecks), and incentives (e.g., weight loss starter kit). All staff should be properly trained to answer questions regarding the weight loss program, and the clinic may also host events involving current weight loss clients and to advertise to new clients. These may include regular group walks, clinic-sponsored community walks, or fun runs, and can act as the support sessions provided for owners embarking on their weight loss journey. For feline owners, consider the establishment of a cat activity area (see Box 8.2 for an example cat activity area).

BOX 8.2: Special focus on Bug's Cat Gym

Kenneth J. Lambrecht

GENESIS

The development of Bug's Cat Gym started following publication of data showing ideal weight dogs live almost 2 years longer than their overweight counterparts (1). When moving to a new location, the owner of a Midwestern veterinary facility applied this information to the development and design of the new space with a focus on ideal weight and nutrition. The portion dedicated to cats was also designed to meet the requirements to become designated a gold level Cat Friendly Practice per the American Association of Feline Practitioners.

CREATING THE EQUIPMENT AND REFINING THE SPACE

The clinic started with two cat walks connected by tunnels above the reception area (Figure 8.2) and then added a full gym and boarding area for cats on the second story of the building (Figure 8.3). "Bug Mountain" became the first piece designed for this cat-friendly space. It was made out of two pieces of plywood with holes cut for interior cat access and hiding spaces below. It was angled to allow for vertical climbing and escape (Figure 8.4). A stone climbing wall and One Fast Cat exercise wheel (2) were added next. The practice then created "Bug's Private Gym" for shy boarding cats to exercise with access to private condos via tunnels (Figure 8.5). More climbing perches and elevated cat walkways were added, allowing cats to be above the action for the full circumference of the room (Figure 8.6).

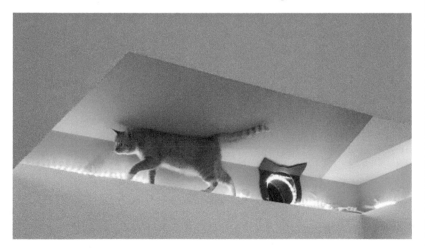

Figure 8.2 Reception cat walks. Two cat walks connected by tunnels were placed above the hospital reception area. (Used with permission from the West Towne Veterinary Center, Madison, Wisconsin.)

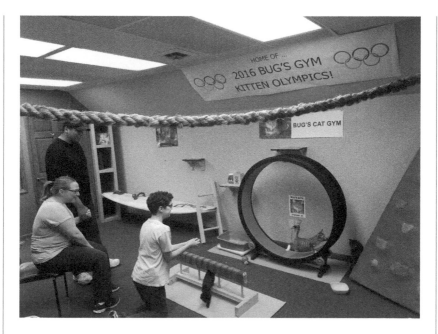

Figure 8.3 Bug's Cat Gym. Full gym and boarding area for cats on the second story of the building. (Used with permission from the West Towne Veterinary Center, Madison, Wisconsin.)

"PETS REDUCING FOR RESCUES" IDEAL WEIGHT MANAGEMENT PROGRAMS AND "CAT'S NIGHT OUT"

Bug's Cat Gym is an integral part of the clinic's annual 8-week Pets Reducing for Rescues (PRFR) contest. During the contest, local pet owners and rescues enter overweight cats to participate in a weight management program. Every pound lost by the cats results in a donation to a local rescue from the clinic, part of which is defrayed by the sale of products donated by corporate sponsors. Participation incentives include door prizes available during the initial weigh-in, as well as opportunities to purchase activity monitors, scales and automated feeders at a discounted price, with proceeds donated to participating rescue organizations. PRFR cats gain access to the gym via scheduled appointments, on an individual basis if they are new or shy, or via monthly "Cat's Night Out" events. These events include educational discussions on proper feeding and exercise, specific to the behavioral aspects of cats. Cat owners who have successfully participated in a weight loss program help manage these events and provide support for those just starting on a weight loss journey with their cats. Bug's Cat Gym serves to make weight loss more fun for both the cats and the people. The clinic has also found the cats typically become much more social and lively with repeated exposure to the gym and participation in the monthly Cat's Night Out events.

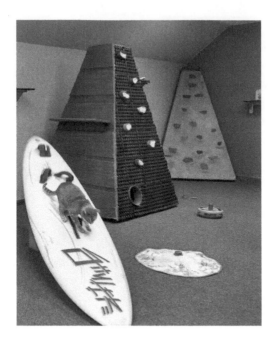

Figure 8.4 Bug's Mountain. Bug's Mountain consists of two pieces of plywood with holes cut for interior cat access and hiding spaces below. It is angled to allow for vertical climbing and escape. A stone climbing wall is also visible in the background. (Used with permission from the West Towne Veterinary Center, Madison, Wisconsin.)

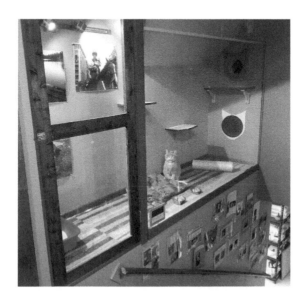

Figure 8.5 Bug's Private Gym. (Used with permission from the West Towne Veterinary Center, Madison, Wisconsin.)

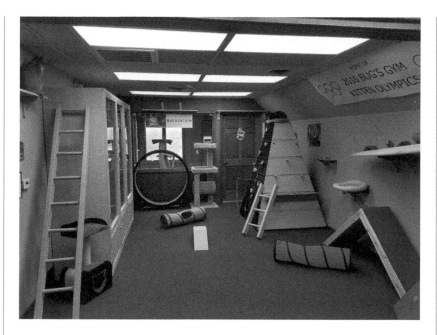

Figure 8.6 More climbing perches and elevated cat walkways were added, allowing cats to be above the action for the full circumference of the room. (Used with permission from the West Towne Veterinary Center, Madison, Wisconsin.)

REFERENCES

1. Kealy RD, Lawler DF, Ballam JM et al. Effects of diet restriction on life span and age-related changes in dogs. *Journal of the American Veterinary Medical Association* 2002;220(9):1315–1320.
2. One Fast Cat. Cat Exercise Wheel. Available from: http://onefastcat.com. Accessed March 1, 2016.

Collaborative efforts between a rehabilitation/sports medicine facility with qualified personnel (e.g., Diplomate of the American College of Veterinary Sports Medicine and Rehabilitation [DACVSMR], Certified Canine Rehabilitation Practitioner [CCRP], or Certified Canine Rehabilitation Therapist [CCRT]) can be used to further achieve success with a weight loss program (see Chapter 7). If not affiliated with one's own hospital, a cooperative referral system can be established between facilities. If rehabilitation or exercise services are available within a single hospital network, assessment by the rehabilitation/sports medicine service for exercise recommendations may be included as part of the initial weight loss evaluation. Alternatively, weight loss assessment can be recommended for any patient primarily consulting with rehabilitation/sports medicine services that is also overweight or obese. Contact with local pet agility or dock diving organizations is another opportunity to provide owners with resources to encourage interaction with their pets via activity rather than feeding. Some of these organizations may be interested in cosponsoring an event geared toward obese or overweight pets just starting out.

There may also be opportunities within the community to work together with human weight loss clinics, dietitians, or gym facilities with expertise in weight loss programs for people. Consider offering veterinary support to these facilities, focusing on overweight people who also have overweight pets.

8.5.1 Quick tips

- Prepare marketing materials to provide to owners (in clinic and online).
- Train all staff to properly answer questions regarding a weight loss program.
- Consider hosting events to promote weight loss or healthy body weight to support existing clients, but also advertise to new clients.
- Identify a local animal rehabilitation/sports medicine program with qualified personnel to establish collaborative referral efforts or establish cooperative services within one's own hospital.
- Contact local organizations such as agility or dock diving groups to provide additional resources for exercise to owners.
- Offer veterinary services to local human weight loss facilities, focusing on overweight owners who also have overweight pets.

8.6 THE FINANCIAL IMPLICATIONS

Financial constraints may impede an owner's willingness to participate in a weight loss program for their pet. Paying a full consultation fee every 2–4 weeks during a weight loss program, likely to take 6–12 months or even longer (20), will be out of reach for many pet owners. Those with medical insurance for their pets may fare better, but some policies may not include benefits related to weight loss programs. For this reason, the clinic should consider offering some or all weight checks free of charge by utilizing veterinary nurse appointments, creating discounted weight recheck appointment fees, or instead charging an obesity consultation package fee. Exactly what is included within such a package can be decided by the practice, but options include any or all of the following:

1. Weight checks alone with veterinarian and/or nurse
2. Weight loss food (or a discount voucher)
3. Gram scales (if provided)
4. Rewards and incentives
5. Routine laboratory testing (e.g., periodic CBC, chemistry panel and urinalysis)
6. Access to online resources
7. A follow-up weight maintenance program

Practices could consider offering a variety of packages with different costs, so as to enable a client to choose the option that suits them. Rather than weight loss packages, weight management "bundles" could be an alternative (e.g., an upfront fee covering a designated number of weight recheck appointments). After these rechecks are redeemed, additional appointments can be paid for individually, further bundles purchased, or the client could transition to a formal weight management package. In people, 95% of those who completed a 2-year lifestyle-based weight loss program reported willingness to pay for continued weight loss interventions involving monthly coaching contact (23).

From a financial and marketing perspective, the clinic may consider setting the package as a loss leader for the hospital (24). Although it may be counterintuitive, allowing a slight financial loss for weight management services may encourage the owner to commit to the weight loss program, and then engage in regular visits to the hospital. Not only does this help to bond the client with the practice, but more frequent visits to the hospital will likely benefit the practice through increased sales (e.g., renewing prescriptions, scheduling wellness appointments, purchasing preventatives). Finally, such weight loss checks might enable early identification of other diseases, which then require follow-up at the clinic.

As with any new program or service introduced to the clinic, a cost-benefit analysis should be performed prior to setting the final client fee. This process involves developing a list of benefits to the clinic compared to the financial cost of implementation. Benefits may be tangible (e.g., clinic revenue) or nontangible (e.g., client word of mouth, media attention, hospital advertising when patient wears branded bandana/leash/collar). One of the larger costs to the clinic may be the weight loss starter kit or incentive rewards. Methods to reduce the cost of this kit include purchasing items in bulk, obtaining item donations, and requesting food samples or coupons from pet food manufacturers.

Implementation of a system including discounted weight recheck appointments may pose a challenge for the general practice setting if owners schedule these visits with the goal of actually discussing the pet's newly developed, and unrelated, medical problem. Client communication is key in this regard from all those conversing with the client when scheduling and then participating in the weight recheck appointment. Hospital staff should always refer to the booking as a weight recheck appointment and consider reiterating that it does not include a full physical examination. Hospital staff likely to interact with these pet owners includes:

1. The client services representative who books the appointment
2. The client services representative who greets the owner when checking in for their appointment
3. The veterinary nurse or assistant who either loads the pet for the attending veterinarian or completes the weight recheck
4. The attending veterinarian who evaluates the pet (if the session is not completed by the veterinary nurse)
5. The client services representative who checks the patient out of the hospital after their visit

These staff members are encouraged to refer to the visits as weight loss or maintenance program visits in order to reduce any client confusion regarding their expected scope.

8.6.1 Quick tips

- Consider charging a discounted weight recheck appointment fee and/or creating a bundled weight loss program and recheck appointment package.
- Consider creating the program as a loss leader for the hospital.
- A cost-benefit analysis should be used to determine the program benefit versus the cost of implementation.
- All staff involved with these appointments must clearly communicate they are weight recheck or maintenance appointments and do not include general wellness or ill-pet full physical examination.

8.7 CONCLUSION

Each veterinary clinic establishing a weight management program should first create resources to help the client and pet achieve weight loss and eventual ideal weight maintenance as efficiently as possible. An initial information questionnaire (DAHHF), treat allowance sheets, weekly food diary, and clearly illustrated ideal weight and BCS goals will help the veterinary staff and owner communicate about feeding recommendations. Before and after pet pictures, weight loss starter kits, and certificates of weight loss completion can help incentivize owners and maintain commitment to program compliance. Compliance is also fostered via consistent recheck appointments and open access to clinic scales for owners to check their pet's progress between scheduled weight assessments. Clear feeding instructions to aid ideal weight maintenance and continued weight rechecks at least every 6 months should be sustained long term. Marketing materials and hospital events related to weight loss can serve as program advertisement to the community, as can collaboration with other veterinary or human medical professionals. Finally, financial costs involved with establishing a weight management program should be assessed via a cost-benefit analysis to ensure the program is realistic and sustainable from both the client and clinic perspective.

APPENDIX 8.1: DIET, ACTIVITY, AND HOUSEHOLD HISTORY FORM

The following example form is based on those in use at the University of Liverpool Royal Canin Weight Management Clinic and the University of Tennessee College of Veterinary Medicine Nutrition Service.

Pet information questionnaire for new cases

The main aim of this questionnaire is to provide us with preliminary information about your pet, prior to you visiting the clinic. We will use this questionnaire to form the basis of the consultation. It will also allow us to tailor an appropriate weight management regime for your pet's circumstances.

Please consult all family members (if possible), and answer the questions as honestly as possible. If you are uncertain of the meaning of any particular question, don't worry; we can clarify this during your visit. Also, if you would prefer not to answer any question, please feel free to leave it blank.

Section 1: About your pet

Pet's Name: _____ Surname/Last Name: _____

Species: ☐ Canine ☐ Feline   Sex/status: ☐ Intact Female ☐ Spayed Female

                                                    ☐ Intact Male ☐ Neutered Male

Breed: _____ Date of Birth: _____ Age: _____ (Years / Months)

What age was your pet neutered? _____

Where did your pet come from (e.g., breeder, rescue, shelter)? _____

      How old was your pet at that time? Age: _____ (Years / Months / Weeks)

When was your pet last vaccinated? _____

Please let us know of any illness your pet has suffered in the last 12 months:

_____

_____

_____

_____

_____

Please let us know of any other previous medical concerns for your pet:

_____

_____

_____

_____

Is your animal insured? ☐ Yes ☐ No

      If yes, with whom? _____

Have you noticed any change in your pet's urination? ☐ Yes ☐ No

    If YES, please describe: _____

_____

Have you noticed any change in your pet's defecation? ☐ Yes ☐ No

    If YES, please describe: _____

_____

Does your pet currently have a good appetite? ☐ Yes ☐ No

    If NO, please describe: _____

_____

Has your pet's appetite recently changed? ☐ Yes ☐ No

    If YES, please describe: _____

_____

Has your pet experienced any undesired weight gain or weight loss? ☐ Yes ☐ No

    If YES, please describe: _____

_____

What is your pet's current weight? _____ ☐ Pounds ☐ Kilograms   Date measured: _____

Is your pet: ☐ Underweight ☐ Ideal Weight ☐ Overweight

    If over- or underweight, what is your pet's ideal weight? _____ ☐ Pounds ☐ Kilograms

Current Flea/Tick/Heartworm Prevention (name and frequency of administration):

    EXAMPLE: Brand X Flea Control (for 10 – 22 pound dogs): 1 chew every 4 weeks (last given 10/1/2018)

    1. _____
    2. _____
    3. _____

Current Medications/Supplements (name and dose per day):

    EXAMPLE: Prednisone (5 mg tablets): 1 ½ tablets twice daily

    1. _____
    2. _____
    3. _____
    4. _____
    5. _____
    6. _____
    7. _____
    8. _____

Section 2: About your family

Please provide details of everyone who lives in your household

	Age	Gender	Relation	Occupation
You				
Others				

Please complete below if required

Please describe any care not provided by the primary owners (e.g., day care, dog walker, boarding, pet sitter):

_____

_____

_____

Please provide details of your other pets

Name	Species	Breed	Age	Gender	Neutered (Y/N)	Related (Y/N)

Please complete below if required

The remaining questions are to be completed for the pet who will be attending the clinic

Section 3: Feeding and Treating

Who feeds this pet? _____

Where is your pet typically fed (e.g., kitchen, laundry room, kennel, outside)? _____

How many meals (food put into a bowl) does your pet have on a normal day?

☐ One ☐ Two ☐ Three ☐ Four ☐ Left out ☐ Other: _____

Is your pet fed from the same bowl as other pets in the house? ☐ Yes ☐ No

    If YES, please describe: _____

Is there competition for food between pets? ☐ Yes ☐ No

    If YES, please describe: _____

Does your pet have access to food other than its own? ☐ Yes ☐ No

    If YES, please describe: _____

Does your pet ever gain access to the trash? ☐ Yes ☐ No

    If YES, how often does your pet get into the trash? _____

Complete Diet History: (Commercially Available Diets)

Diet Type	Brand	Flavor	Amount Fed Per Meal	Times Fed Per Day	Fed Since or Dates Fed	Reason Stopped

Please complete below if required

Complete Diet History: (Home Prepared Diets)

Diet/Ingredient Type	Preparation Method	Amount Fed Per Meal	Times Fed Per Day	Fed Since or Dates Fed	Reason Stopped

Please complete below if required

Complete Treat History: (Commercially Available Treats, Chews, Etc.)

Treat Type	Brand	Flavor	Size	Number Fed Per Day	Fed Since or Dates Fed	Reason Stopped

Please complete below if required

Complete Treat History: (Human Food Treats, Table Scraps, Left Overs, Etc.)

Treat Type	Ingredient	Serving Size	Times Fed Per Day	Fed Since or Dates Fed	Reason Stopped

Please complete below if required

Do you use food/treats to administer medications or supplements? ☐ Yes ☐ No

    If YES, please describe: _____

What does your pet drink?

    ☐ Tap water ☐ Well water ☐ Bottled water ☐ Milk ☐ Tea ☐ Other: _____

How do you measure out your pet's food?

    ☐ Estimate amount ☐ Measuring cup / scoop ☐ Weigh on a scale ☐ Other: _____

Does your pet ask for food? ☐ Yes ☐ No

    If your pet asks for food, how often does he/she do this?

        ☐ All day   ☐ Several times a day ☐ Once or twice a day ☐ Less than once a day

Section 4: Environment - Dogs

On a scale of 1 – 10 how active is your dog? _____

    1 = Very inactive. Sleeps the majority of the day. Rarely playful when exercised.

    10 = Very Active. Thoroughly enjoys exercise, often active inside or out.

How often do you exercise your dog?

    ☐ More than once per day ☐ Once per day ☐ Some days ☐ None ☐ Other: _____

Where do you exercise your dog?

    ☐ House/apartment on one level   ☐ House apartment on more than one level (i.e., stairs)

    ☐ Back yard   ☐ Garden   ☐ Local pavement walks   ☐ Local park/play area

    ☐ Country parks   ☐ Fields or woodland ☐ Dog park   ☐ Other: _____

On average, how long is your dog exercised at each session?

    ☐ 10 minutes or less ☐ 10 – 20 minutes   ☐ 20 – 60 minutes   ☐ 1 hour or more

    ☐ Other: _____

During exercise sessions, does your dog

    ☐ Play with the walker   ☐ Play with ball/stick/other toys   ☐ Go off lead

    ☐ Walk on extendable/retractable lead   ☐ Other: _____

Where do you and your dog live?

    ☐ Apartment with a yard/garden   ☐ Apartment without a yard/garden

    ☐ House with a yard/garden   ☐ House without a yard/garden

    ☐ Bungalow with a yard/garden   ☐ Bungalow without a yard/garden

    ☐ Other: _____

Where does your dog spend most of its time?

    ☐ Indoors   ☐ Outdoors   ☐ Both indoors & outdoors

Does your dog have access to the outdoors?

    ☐ No   ☐ Fenced yard/garden ☐ Unfenced yard/garden   ☐ Lead walks only

How much time does your dog spend outdoors?

    Weekdays _____ Weekends _____

How many hours per day is your dog left alone?

    ☐ 0 – 2 hours   ☐ 2 – 5 hours   ☐ 5 – 8 hours   ☐ 8+ hours

On a scale of 1 – 10 how well trained is your dog? _____

    1 = Untrained (no basic obedience)

    10 = Highly trained (e.g., agility trained, show dog, tricks)

Section 4: Environment - Cats

On a scale of 1 – 10 how active is your cat? _____

    1 = Very inactive. Rarely, if ever exercises. Does the minimum necessary.

    10 = Very Active. Frequently exercised, always on the go, very energetic when playing.

Where does your cat spend most of its time?

☐ Indoors   ☐ Outdoors   ☐ Both indoors & outdoors

Does your cat have restricted access to the outdoors? ☐ Yes ☐ No

    If yes, when do you confine your cat to the house?

        ☐ During the night   ☐ When owners are at work

        ☐ During the day when owners are home   ☐ Other: _____

How much time does your cat spend outside per day?

☐ Less than 1 hour   ☐ 1 – 3 hours   ☐ 3 – 6 hours   ☐ 6+ hours

Does your cat hunt? ☐ Yes ☐ No

    Does your cat bring back live prey? ☐ Yes ☐ No

How many hours per day is your cat left alone?

☐ 0 – 2 hours   ☐ 2 – 5 hours   ☐ 5 – 8 hours   ☐ 8+ hours

Does your cat ever hide within the home? ☐ Yes ☐ No

    If YES, where does the cat hide? _____

Does your cat play on its own? ☐ Yes ☐ No

    If YES, how often?   ☐ Once per day   ☐ More than once per day

        ☐ Once a week   ☐ More than once a week   ☐ Less than once a week

Do you play with your cat?   ☐ Yes ☐ No

    If YES, how often?   ☐ Once per day   ☐ More than once per day

        ☐ Once a week   ☐ More than once a week   ☐ Less than once a week

What kind of toys does your cat prefer?

☐ Balls   ☐ Fishing toys   ☐ Rolled up newspaper   ☐ Clockwork toys

☐ Catnip   ☐ Other: _____

How many hours per day does your cat sleep?   ☐ Less than 12 hours   ☐ More than 12 hours

Where do you and your cat live?

☐ Apartment with a yard/garden   ☐ Apartment without a yard/garden

☐ House with a yard/garden   ☐ House without a yard/garden

☐ Bungalow with a yard/garden   ☐ Bungalow without a yard/garden

☐ Other: _____

If you have more than one cat in your household, which of the following resources do the cats share?

☐ Feeding stations   ☐ Water stations   ☐ Resting places   ☐ Litter trays

APPENDIX 8.2: CLIENT PHOTOGRAPH RELEASE CONSENT FORM

This release form should be signed by the owner at the initial appointment if photographs of their pet may be used for marketing or displayed to the public. (This form adapted and used with permission from the Red Bank Veterinary Hospital, Tinton Falls, New Jersey.)

I, _____ , hereby grant permission to the

_____(Hospital Name)_____ to use my pet's medical story, my own image and my

pet's image in perpetuity, in any media, now known or hereinafter devised, and I

acknowledge the right to alter said image(s) at their discretion. I also acknowledge that

they may choose not to use these images or my pet's medical story at this time, but may do

so at their discretion at a later date. The _____(Hospital Name)_____ also reserves the

right to discontinue use of said images without notice. I understand that if my own image

or my pet's image is used, published or posted on the _____(Hospital Name)_____

website, the image is available to be downloaded by any computer user. Therefore, I agree

to indemnify and hold harmless from any claims arising from use of said images, the staff

employed by _____(Hospital Name)_____ .

_____

Signature

_____

Date

_____

(Hospital Name) Representative

APPENDIX 8.3: TREAT ALLOWANCE SHEETS

Cat and dog daily treat allowance sheets are tailored to the individual patient. Both current treats and a few low calorie treats recommended by the clinic should be included to help owners clearly see how they are utilizing their treat allowance and to avoid providing excess treat calories. (These examples are modified with permission from the University of Tennessee College of Veterinary Medicine Nutrition Service.)

DAILY TREAT ALLOWANCE - CATS

Name: _____ Maximum calories per day: _____

To maintain a well-balanced diet, treats should not exceed more than ten percent of total daily caloric intake. You may mix and match the treats below as long as you do not exceed the recommended maximum calories per day. The treats listed below are not an endorsement of a particular manufacturer or guarantee of results.

Current Treats

This list is based on treats you are currently feeding. If you wish to feed additional treats, please consider caloric content of individual products to ensure you are not exceeding your pet's recommended daily treat allowance.

Brand/Product Name	Calories per treat

Low Calorie Commercial Treats

The calorie content of the following treats generally allow for feeding multiple pieces per day within a daily allowance.

Brand/Product Name	Calories per treat
Brand X Crunchy Cat Treats – any flavor	1.1
Brand X Dental Treats – any flavor	1.25
Brand X Dental Cat Treats	1.3
Brand X Cat Treats – any flavor	1.5
Brand X Treats for cats – any flavor	2
Brand X Treats Chicken & Potato Formula	3

Treat Dispensing Toys

The toys listed below may be useful to increase your cat's daily activity. The treat allotment, or a portion of the daily meal, may be placed inside these toys to encourage healthy environmental stimulation for your cat.

Brand/Product Name
Brand X Tunnel Feeder Cat Toy
Brand X Cat Toy
Brand X Cat Treat Cone
Brand X Interactive Cat Toy

Date Last Updated: _____

DAILY TREAT ALLOWANCE - DOGS

Name: _____ Maximum calories per day: _____

To maintain a well-balanced diet, treats should not exceed more than ten percent of total daily caloric intake. You may mix and match the treats below as long as you do not exceed the recommended maximum calories per day. The treats listed below are not an endorsement of a particular manufacturer or guarantee of results.

Current Treats

This list is based on treats you are currently feeding. If you wish to feed additional treats, please consider caloric content of individual products to ensure you are not exceeding your pet's recommended daily treat allowance.

Brand/Product Name	Treat Size	Calories per treat

Low Calorie Commercial Treats

The calorie content of the following treats generally allow for feeding multiple pieces per day within a daily allowance.

Brand/Product Name	Treat Size	Calories per treat
Brand X Baked Treats	Extra Small	4
Brand X Cheese Flavored Treats	Mini	4.5
Brand X Crunchy Treats – Any flavor	Small	6
Brand X Chewy Treats	Small	9
Brand X Soft-Baked Treats	One Size	12
Brand X Biscuits	Medium	20

Dental Commercial Treats (Veterinary Oral Health Council Seal)

The treats listed below are recognized to slow the build-up of plaque and tartar, when given as described on the product label. *Please note: your pet's treat allowance may be lower than the caloric content of many dental treat options.*

Brand/Product Name	Treat Size	Calories per treat
Brand X Dental Treats	Extra Small	26
Brand X Oral Care Dental Treats	Small	63
Brand X Minty Breath Dental Treats	Large	99

Date Last Updated: _____

APPENDIX 8.4: WEEKLY FOOD DIARY

This allows owners to record food offered, food consumed, activity, "confessions" (e.g., occasions when additional food has been consumed, be it stolen by the animal or given by the owner as a treat), demeanor, and any other observations (such as other illnesses). (Modified with permission from the University of Liverpool Royal Canin Weight Management Clinic, Neston, United Kingdom.)

Weekly food diary

Name: _____

Date	Food given	Food eaten (All/half/none)	Exercise How much/how often?	General observations	Confessions	Concerns/comments

Number of weeks on diet

• Please indicate when a new bag, tray, can, pouch or box of food is started

_____

REFERENCES

1. Murphy M. Obesity treatment: Environment and behavior modification. *Veterinary Clinics of North America: Small Animal Practice* 2016;46:883–898.
2. Linder D, Mueller M. Pet obesity management: Beyond nutrition. *Veterinary Clinics of North America: Small Animal Practice* 2014;44: 789–806, vii.
3. German AJ, Holden SL, Gernon LJ et al. Do feeding practices of obese dogs, before weight loss, affect the success of weight management? *British Journal of Nutrition* 2011;106 (Suppl 1):S97–S100.
4. German AJ, Holden SL, Wiseman-Orr ML et al. Quality of life is reduced in obese dogs but improves after successful weight loss. *Veterinary Journal* 2012;192:428–434.
5. German AJ, Holden SL, Morris PJ et al. Long-term follow-up after weight management in obese dogs: The role of diet in preventing regain. *Veterinary Journal* 2012;192:65–70.

6. Deagle G, Holden SL, Biourge V et al. Long-term follow-up after weight management in obese cats. *Journal of Nutritional Science* 2014;3:e25.

7. Schoeller DA. Limitations in the assessment of dietary energy intake by self-report. *Metabolism* 1995;44:18–22.

8. Archer E, Pavela G, Lavie CJ. The inadmissibility of what we eat in America and NHANES dietary data in nutrition and obesity research and the scientific formulation of national dietary guidelines. *Mayo Clinic Proceedings* 2015;90:911–926.

9. Laflamme D. Development and validation of a body condition score system for cats: A clinical tool. *The Feline Practice* 1997;25:13–17.

10. Laflamme DP. Development and validation of a body condition score system for dogs. *Canine Practice* 1997;1997:10–15.

11. Thatcher CD, Hand MS, Remillard RL. Small animal clinical nutrition: An iterative process. In: *Small Animal Clinical Nutrition*, 5th ed., MS Hand, CD Thatcher, RL Remillard et al. (eds.). Topeka, KS: Mark Morris Institute; 2010, pp. 3–21.

12. German AJ, Holden SL, Moxham GL et al. A simple, reliable tool for owners to assess the body condition of their dog or cat. *Journal of Nutrition* 2006;136:2031S–2033S.

13. World Small Animal Veterinary Association Global Nutrition Committee. Body condition score chart dogs. 2013. Available at: http://www.wsava.org/sites/default/files/Body%20condition%20score%20chart%20dogs.pdf. Accessed February 28, 2016.

14. World Small Animal Veterinary Association Global Nutrition Committee. Body condition score chart cats. 2013. Available from: http://www.wsava.org/sites/default/files/Body%20condition%20score%20chart%20cats.pdf. Accessed February 28, 2016.

15. German A, Heath S. Feline obesity: A medical disease with behavioral consequences. In: *Feline Behavioral Health and Welfare*, 1st ed., I Rodan, S Heath (eds.). St. Louis, MO: Saunders; 2015, pp. 148–161.

16. American Animal Hospital Association. Compliance: Taking quality care to the next level: A report of the 2009 AAHA compliance follow-up study; 2009:18. Available from: https://secure.aahanet.org/eweb/images/student/pdf/Compliance.pdf.

17. National Heart, Lung, and Blood Institute with The National Institute of Diabetes and Digestive and Kidney Diseases. *Clinical Guidelines on the Identification, Evaluation, and Treatment of Overweight and Obesity in Adults: The Evidence Report.* Publication No. 98-4083. Bethesda, MD: National Institutes of Health, National Heart, Lung, and Blood, Institute; 1998.

18. German AJ, Holden SL, Bissot T et al. Use of starting condition score to estimate changes in body weight and composition during weight loss in obese dogs. *Research in Veterinary Science* 2009;87:249–254.

19. Baker SG, Roush JK, Unis MD et al. Comparison of four commercial devices to measure limb circumference in dogs. *Veterinary and Comparative Orthopaedics and Traumatology* 2010;23:406–410.

20. German AJ, Titcomb JM, Holden SL et al. Cohort study of the success of controlled weight loss programs for obese dogs. *Journal of Veterinary Internal Medicine* 2015;29:1547–1555.
21. German AJ, Holden SL, Mason SL et al. Imprecision when using measuring cups to weigh out extruded dry kibbled food. *Journal of Animal Physiology and Animal Nutrition* 2011;95:368–373.
22. Murphy M, Lusby AL, Bartges JW et al. Size of food bowl and scoop affects amount of food owners feed their dogs. *Journal of Animal Physiology and Animal Nutrition* 2012;96:237–241.
23. Jerome GJ, Alavi R, Daumit GL et al. Willingness to pay for continued delivery of a lifestyle-based weight loss program: The Hopkins POWER trial. *Obesity* 2015;23:282–285.
24. Hess J, Gerstner E. Loss leader pricing and rain check policy. *Marketing Science* 1987;6:358–374.

9

Case Examples

9.1 CASE 1: SUCCESSFUL WEIGHT LOSS AND WEIGHT MAINTENANCE IN A DACHSHUND FOLLOWING INTERVERTEBRAL DISK HERNIATION SURGERY: THE IMPORTANCE OF RISK FACTOR ASSESSMENT

MORAN TAL, CLAUDIA WONG, AND ADRONIE VERBRUGGHE

9.1.1 Patient history

A 6-year-old male, neutered dachshund presented for back pain. Magnetic resonance imaging revealed a cervical disc compression of the spinal cord between C5 and C6, and a ventral slot corpectomy was performed. As the patient was assessed as obese by the institution's neurology service, weight loss was recommended to reduce joint stress, and the patient's owners consented to pursuing weight loss with the institution's clinical nutrition service.

9.1.2 Patient assessment

Upon the nutrition consult (time point will be referred to as T0), the patient was recovering well. The only abnormality on nutritional screening evaluation, performed according to the World Small Animal Veterinary Association nutritional assessment guidelines (1), was obesity. At presentation, he was fed a pet store brand dry dog food* for all life stages twice daily (pet food label information: metabolizable energy [ME] 478 kcal/cup or 3900 kcal/kg, and values were calculated from the guaranteed analysis; 108.2 g/1000 kcal protein [min]; 51.3 g/1000 kcal fat [min]; 14.1 g/1000 kcal crude fiber [max]). An accurate daily energy intake could not be calculated because his food was being measured using a recycled container, where two full containers were measured by the owners to be slightly less than one standard cup (8 oz, 250 mL). The dog was fed two containers a day. Additionally, he received cooked chicken (~112 kcal/4 tbsp or 60 g daily)

---

* Orijen, Original Dog Food (dry), Edmonton, Canada.

with meals to stimulate his interest in food, and commercial treats for which no caloric information was available. Smoked beef marrow bone (~198 kcal/96 g of 1 bone) and raw vegetables were also given throughout the day. Overall, more than 37.5% (>300 kcal/day) of his daily caloric intake originated from treats and unbalanced table food.

His body condition score (BCS) (2) was assessed as 9/9 (approximately 50% body fat, estimated according to clinician's experience), but the muscle condition score (MCS) (3) could not be assessed due to too much fat coverage. His initial body weight (BW) was 15.8 kg, while his estimated ideal BW was calculated to be 9.88 kg ([15.8 kg × 50% lean mass]/80% lean mass) (2,4).

As the patient presented with a BCS larger than 5/9, an extended nutritional evaluation was indicated (1). Animal factors contributing to obesity in this patient include dachshund breed, neutered male, and middle age. Dietary factors include a high energy density diet, feeding excessive treats and human foods, and poor measurement of meals. Last, the patient also had a low activity level, especially because of the recent recovery period.

9.1.3 Plan

A veterinary therapeutic diet formulated for weight loss,* dry and canned formulas (nutrient compositions for dry and canned food, respectively: ME 360 kcal/100 g and 56 kcal/100 g; 94.4 and 121.8 g/1000 kcal protein; 27.8 and 35.8 g/1000 kcal fat; 7.5 and 17.9 g/1000 kcal crude fiber; 83.3 and 62.7 g/1000 kcal L-carnitine) were selected out of several options. The daily energy intake was calculated based on an ideal body weight of 9.88 kg to be 390 kcal/day using a maintenance energy requirement (MER) factor of 1.0 for weight loss (MER = $70 \times [9.88]^{0.75} \times 1.0 = 390$ kcal/day) (4).

The dog was fed three meals per day to increase satiety and reduce begging behavior. His owners were encouraged to feed him using feeding toys (puzzles and kong†) for enrichment and to increase activity. For treats, low-calorie, veterinary therapeutic dog biscuits‡ (ME 15 kcal/treat) and raw vegetables were recommended, not exceeding 10% of daily energy intake, to maintain a balanced nutrient profile (5). All other treats and human foods were strictly prohibited. The owners were instructed to weigh each meal using a kitchen gram scale to ensure accurate feeding amounts. To ensure a slow and consistent weight loss of 1%–2% per week (6), where 2% is the recommended maximum amount of safe weight loss (4), biweekly weigh-ins were recommended, always using the same scale at the family veterinarian's practice. According to the literature, if the weight change is lower than 0.5%, a reduction range of 5%–20% of daily energy intake is recommended (4,7), therefore, the food amount was adjusted as required based on weight loss.

---

* Royal Canin Veterinary Diets, Canine Calorie Control (dry and canned), Ontario, Canada.
† The Kong Company, Golden, Colorado.
‡ Purina Pro Plan Veterinary Diets, Lite Snackers, Ontario, Canada.

9.1.4 Short- and long-term follow-up

Twelve days after T0, 0.9 kg weight loss (average of 3.5% per week) was reported (BW 14 kg), and food intake adjustments were considered for a more gradual weight loss, if this rate continued. Ten days later, his BW remained unchanged. The diet plan was adjusted and the daily energy intake was reduced to 360 kcal/day (8% decrease) and divided into four meals per day instead of three. Following this adjustment, steady weight loss resumed further for 4 more weeks and then plateaued.

Two months (68 days) after T0, the patient and owner came in for a recheck appointment (Figure 9.1). Although recent weight trends showed a plateau, the dog's body condition had improved from a 9/9 BCS to an 8/9 (BW 12.2 kg). Improvements of mobility and energy level were reported by the owners, and the owners were recommended to continue the same course. However, at the next weight update, 13 days after the recheck, the patient gained 0.2 kg. With the warming weather, the owners believed they could increase the dog's activity level, so changes were again postponed until the next update.

As predicted, with increased exercise (e.g., increased number and duration of daily walks) the dog continued to lose weight steadily through the spring. The rate of weight loss varied; however, approximately 6 months after T0, the dog reached a BW of 10.0 kg.

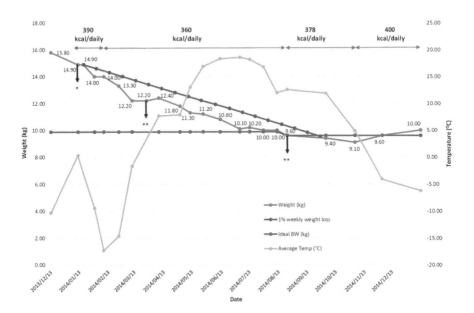

Figure 9.1 Weight loss trends (blue) plotted against ideal body weight (purple), an average weekly weight loss of 1% of the initial body weight (red), and average temperatures (green). Caloric intake over time is presented at the top of the graph (orange). *January 17, 2014: Start of weight loss plan (T0); **March 26, 2014, and August 22, 2014 (Tm): Recheck appointment.

At the next recheck appointment (7 months after T0), the dog lost an additional 0.4 kg (Figure 9.1), and was assessed to be at ideal BCS and MCS at 9.6 kg. A long-term weight maintenance plan was calculated (time point will be referred to as Tm), using the same two diets, with an increase of the daily energy intake by 5% to 378 kcal/day (4). Monthly weight updates were advised.

A month and a half later, the dog had lost 0.5 kg over two weight updates, so his weight maintenance plan was revised accordingly to a daily energy intake of 400 kcal/day, a 6% increase.

Four months after Tm, the patient had gained 0.5 kg, and due to continuation of weight gain, his daily energy intake was adjusted back to 378 kcal/day for the remainder of the winter, given his lower activity level. At the time of this report, a year after the start of the weight loss plan, the dog is maintaining his BW at this energy intake.

9.1.5 Discussion

As described in Chapter 1, risk factors for obesity include animal-specific factors and human-specific factors such as dietary factors, physical activity, owner attitudes, and household characteristics. In the case presented, nutritional assessment revealed presence of many of those predisposing factors. The dog was a male, neutered dachshund (predisposed breed) (8,9), who was initially fed an over-the-counter high fat diet, with an inappropriate measuring container (imprecise and inaccurate when weighing out the daily portion size) (10). Moreover owners rewarded the dog with unbalanced foods whenever he presented with a begging behavior or when assumed to lack interest in food. Due to back pain the dog was also inactive, which reduced the dog's energy expenditure. Removing some of these predisposing factors is crucial to initiate weight loss.

When designing a weight loss plan, energy restriction, that is, reducing the daily energy intake, is most important to create a negative energy balance (4,11). To achieve this, a veterinary therapeutic diet formulated for weight loss should be selected, as energy restriction of maintenance diets may provide inadequate amounts of essential nutrients such as protein, essential amino acids, essential fatty acids, minerals, and vitamins. Key nutritional factors for weight loss include but are not limited to reduced energy density, hence reduced fat (4,12); increased total dietary fiber (TDF) content (4,13), which also dilutes energy density and contributes to satiety by slowing gastrointestinal transit time (14); and increased protein (>60 g/1000 kcal for 80% restriction of resting energy requirements) (4,15), which is important for lean body mass maintenance during weight loss (15) and for its significant thermic effect (16). A veterinary therapeutic diet formulated for weight loss was selected, considering key nutritional factors for weight loss as mentioned earlier. Moreover, the diet was also suitable for long-term weight management, as it was considered complete and balanced for adult maintenance based on the recommendations of the Association of American Feed Control Officials (17).

Using food toys for feeding and exercise helps the owners feel actively and positively engaged in the weight loss process. Moreover, promoting daily exercise, especially when the weather is amenable (Figure 9.1) not only enhances weight loss and maintains muscle mass but also strengthens the dog–human relationship (18). Changes in rate of weight loss/gain also demonstrate the importance of regular weight updates, communication with clients, and tailoring the weight loss plan to the patient's individual needs.

KEY LEARNING ISSUES

1. Nutritional assessment is highly important in order to identify and eliminate risk factors of obesity.
2. An individualized weight loss plan should be tailored according to the patient and owner needs.
3. Constant reassessment of the weight loss plan is advised, with frequent monitoring and individualized adjustments based on patient, client, and environmental factors.
4. Client communication is key to ensuring successful long-term weight maintenance and quality of life.

REFERENCES

1. Freeman L, Becvarova I, Cave N et al. WSAVA nutritional assessment guidelines. *Journal of Small Animal Practice* 2011;52(7):385–396.
2. Laflamme DP. Development and validation of a body condition score system for dogs. *Canine Practice* 1997;22(4):10–15.
3. Baldwin K, Bartges J, Buffington T et al. AAHA nutritional assessment guidelines for dogs and cats. *Journal of the American Animal Hospital Association* 2010;46(4):285–296.
4. Brooks D, Churchill J, Fein K et al. 2014 AAHA weight management guidelines for dogs and cats. *Journal of the American Animal Hospital Association* 2014;50(1):1–11.
5. Yaissle JE, Holloway C, Buffington CA. Evaluation of owner education as a component of obesity treatment programs for dogs. *Journal of the American Veterinary Medicine Association* 2004;224(12):1932–1935.
6. Laflamme DP, Kuhlman G. The effect of weight loss regimen on subsequent weight maintenance in dogs. *Nutrition Research* 1995;15(7):1019–1028.
7. Fragua V, Barroeta AC, Manzanilla EG, Codony R, Villaverde C. Evaluation of the use of esterified fatty acid oils enriched in medium-chain fatty acids in weight loss diets for dogs. *Journal of Animal Physiology and Animal Nutrition* 2015;99:48–59.
8. Lund EM, Armstrong PJ, Kirk CA, Klausner JS. Prevalence and risk factors for obesity in adult dogs from private US veterinary practices. *International Journal of Applied Research in Veterinary Medicine* 2006;4(2):177.

9. Edney AT, Smith PM. Study of obesity in dogs visiting veterinary practices in the United Kingdom. *Veterinary Record* 1986;118(14):391–396.

10. German AJ, Holden SL, Mason SL et al. Imprecision when using measuring cups to weigh out extruded dry kibbled food. *Journal of Animal Physiology and Animal Nutrition* 2011;95(3):368–373.

11. German AJ. The growing problem of obesity in dogs and cats. *Journal of Nutrition* 2006;136(7 Suppl):1940S–1946S.

12. Borne AT, Wolfsheimer KJ, Truett AA et al. Differential metabolic effects of energy restriction in dogs using diets varying in fat and fiber content. *Obesity Research* 1996;4(4):337–345.

13. Jackson JR, Laflamme DP, Owens SF. Effects of dietary fiber content on satiety in dogs. *Veterinary Clinical Nutrition* 1997;4:130–134.

14. Jewell D, Toll P. Effects of fiber on food intake in dogs. *Veterinary Clinical Nutrition* 1996;3:115–118.

15. Hannah SS, Laflamme DP. Increased dietary protein spares lean body mass during weight loss in dogs (ABSTRACT). *Journal of Veterinary Internal Medicine* 1998;12:224.

16. Hoenig M, Waldron M, Ferguson D. Effect of a high-and low-carbohydrate diet on respiratory exchange ratio and heat production in lean and obese cats before and after weight loss. *Compendium on Continuing Education for the Practising Veterinarian: North American Edition* 2006;28(4):71.

17. Association of American Feed Control Officials (AAFCO). *2014 Official Publication AAFCO*; 2014.

18. Westgarth C, Christian HE, Christley RM. Factors associated with daily walking of dogs. *BMC Veterinary Research* 2015;11:116.

9.2 CASE 2: MORBID OBESITY IN AN ADULT FEMALE, SPAYED SPRINGER SPANIEL

MEGAN SHEPHERD

9.2.1 Patient history

An 8-year-old female, spayed Springer Spaniel, referred to from here on as "the Spaniel," presented to the veterinary teaching hospital (VTH) orthopedic service for right hind lameness evaluation. At presentation, the spaniel weighed 50.9 kilograms (112 pounds) and had a body condition score (BCS) of 9/9. During the orthopedic exam, the Spaniel developed respiratory distress, attributed to her obese condition and the stress of the exam. The orthopedic exam was discontinued and the Spaniel recovered in an oxygen cage. A nutrition consult was requested by the VTH orthopedic service to help the Spaniel lose weight. Physical rehabilitation was discussed with the owners and had been recommended by the attending orthopedic specialist. However, due to the owners' work schedules and proximity to a physical rehabilitation facility, formal physical rehabilitation was not pursued.

The nutritionist met with the owners to obtain a detailed diet history. In the morning, the first owner fed the Spaniel 1 cup of a dry senior dog food* (374 kcal/cup; fed for 1–2 years) and reported that the Spaniel would eat it only after all of the patient's other food was gone. In addition, the Spaniel was fed one dental treat† (42 kcal/small-medium stick), 1 pepperoni slice (95% fat free; ~10 kcal/slice), and half of a low fat/part skim mozzarella stick (~70 kcal/stick). For lunch the first owner fed 4–5 slices of commercial‡ chicken or turkey. For dinner, the second owner fed 1 cup of the same dry senior dog food and half of a low fat/part skim mozzarella stick (previously, the second owner fed one whole mozzarella stick). Multiple treats were fed when administering medications, kenneling, and when begging between meals. The treats included cooked eggs (2 whole eggs ± 1 egg white per day), potted meat food product (the Spaniel recently stopped eating), baked plain chicken breast, spaghetti, macaroni and cheese, mozzarella cheese sticks (1/2 stick), pepperoni, or more of the dry senior dog food. Table scraps were fed when the owners had leftovers available from their meals. The Spaniel's current diet had been fed for 1–2 years. The nutritionist estimated that the current diet provided a minimum 1300 kcal per day. The owners recently tried feeding a therapeutic weight loss diet§ for 1–2 weeks to promote weight loss. The Spaniel ate the therapeutic weight loss diet initially, but then lost interest.

---

* Exclusive Chicken & Rice Formula Senior Dog Food (374 kcal/cup; kcal/kg information unavailable).
† Pedigree Dentastix Fresh Treats (42 kcal/treat; kcal/kg information unavailable).
‡ Oscar Mayer.
§ Hill's Prescription Diet r/d Canine (dry: 242 kcal/cup, 2968 kcal/kg as fed; canned: 257 kcal/12.3 oz can, 733 kcal/kg as fed).

The owners reported that they did not transition the Spaniel onto the therapeutic weight loss diet.

9.2.2 Patient assessment

Target BCS was set at 5/9. The nutritionist calculated the Spaniel's ideal body weight to be 36.4 kg (80 pounds), based on the assumption that the Spaniel was 140% of ideal body weight ($[50.9 \text{ kg}/140] \times 100 = 36.4 \text{ kg}$) (1). This estimate is likely skewed due to the limits of the 9-point body condition score scale and the chance that the Spaniel was more than 40% above ideal. English Springer Spaniel breed body weight standards are below 50 pounds. The owners were notified that the Spaniel's true ideal body weight would be more accurately determined once an ideal BCS (5/9) had been achieved.

The nutritionist estimated the Spaniel's maintenance energy requirements (MER) to be 1000 kcal per day, based on resting energy requirement (RER; $70 \times 36.4 \text{ kg}^{0.75}$) (1). The goal was for the Spaniel to lose 2–4 kg per month (1%–2% of initial [50.9 kg] body weight per week $= 0.5 - 1$ kg per week). The nutritionist suggested monthly weight rechecks for the duration of the weight loss or at least until a healthy weight loss trend (4–8 pound loss per month) had been established. The nutritionist encouraged the owners to consider using the same scale for each weight recheck. Due to the size of the Spaniel, the floor scale at their local veterinarian's practice was considered most practical.

9.2.3 Plan

The nutritionist set an initial dietary goal to transition the Spaniel onto healthier foods. The nutritionist anticipated that it would take time to get the Spaniel fully transitioned onto healthier foods due to the variety of human foods currently fed. The nutritionist discussed with the owners how it may take up to 4 weeks to get the Spaniel transitioned onto the "ideal" weight loss diet. The nutritionist discussed several therapeutic weight loss diet options, but encouraged the owners to reconsider the original therapeutic weight loss diet, provided it is reintroduced slowly. The owners chose to retry the therapeutic weight loss diet previously fed.

The nutritionist recommended a slow transition onto the therapeutic weight loss diet. It was suggested to take away 1/8–1/4 cup of the dry senior dog food at the Spaniel's breakfast and dinner and replace it with 1/8–1/4 cup of the therapeutic weight loss diet (either dry or canned). Initially and temporarily using flavorful ingredients like tuna juice, canned chicken juice, 1–2 teaspoons of ground beef grease (postcooking), 1 tablespoon of cheese (melted to better stick to the food) or 1 tablespoon parmesan cheese may help with the transition. Alternately, the owners could spread a small amount of the therapeutic weight loss diet canned onto a piece of lunch meat, then slowly spread on more therapeutic weight loss diet canned and reduce the amount of lunch meat.

Once, the Spaniel was transitioned onto the therapeutic weight loss diet, the owners were instructed to follow specific volume guidelines. For the therapeutic weight loss diet, the owners had a choice of either 3.75 cups of the dry kibble,

Table 9.1 Treat options for the Spaniel

Treat item[a]	Amount per day (approximately 100 kcal each)
Broccoli or rainbow slaw	2 cups
Zucchini, raw, sliced	5 cups
Shredded carrots	2 cups
Green beans, boiled, drained, without salt or raw	2 cups
Carrots, baby, boiled, drained, without salt or raw	20 each
Cauliflower boiled, drained, without salt or raw	4 cups
Plain air-popped popcorn (no butter/salt)	3 cups
Part-skim mozzarella, ideally low sodium	1 cheese stick
95% fat free pepperoni, beef or pork, low sodium	10 round slices (max 100 kcal)
Lunch meat (chicken or turkey), low sodium	3–4 slices (check calories per slice, max 100 kcal)
Macaroni, cooked, plain (no sauce)	1/2 cup

[a] The nutrient content of foods was determined using the U.S. Department of Agriculture Nutrient Database (https://ndb.nal.usda.gov/ndb/search).

3.5 cans, or 1.5 cups dry kibble plus 2 cans. The owners were instructed to choose one of the three options per day. The total daily amount of food was to be divided into the three meal times (breakfast, lunch, dinner) per day. Alternately, the owners could divide the food into two meals (breakfast and dinner), then use the recommended treat options during lunch.

Specific treat options were recommended (Table 9.1). Treat allowance was limited to 10% of total daily calories or 100 kcal per day. The owners were informed that the amount recommended for each item met the 10% daily maximum. Therefore, if more than one treat was to be fed per day, the owners were instructed to reduce the amount of each treat respectively. For example, if the owners wanted to feed four treat options (i.e., medication administration, kenneling, and two other between meal times), they were to feed a quarter of the recommended amount for that day.

The nutritionist recommended that the owners encourage voluntary activity. Food toys were discussed as a tool to encourage voluntary movement. Several food toy options were offered* and their use with the dry therapeutic weight loss diet briefly described. The nutritionist encouraged future reconsideration for physical

* KONG Food Toys, Buster Food Cube, Aikiou Activity Food Center, Kyjen Dog Puzzles, Ethical Pet Seek-A-Treat Shuffle Bone Dog Puzzle, StarMark Bob-A-Lot Interactive Pet Toy.

rehabilitation and shared YouTube videos of obese dogs undergoing physical rehabilitation.

The owners were instructed to contact their regular veterinarian in the event of a change in the Spaniel's health status and/or if the Spaniel was losing less than 4 pounds or more than 8 pounds per month. Had the Spaniel lost weight outside of the recommended range, the nutritionist would have rechecked the diet for compliance, then adjusted total daily calories up or down as needed.

9.2.4 Follow-up

At the 4-week phone recheck, the owners reported that the Spaniel was fully transitioned to the therapeutic weight loss diet within the first 4 weeks and that they were seeing a change in the Spaniel's body shape. The owners were pleased with the results thus far. At the 4-month phone recheck, the owners reported that the Spaniel weighed 96 pounds per the scale at the Spaniel's veterinarian's office. The Spaniel was eating the therapeutic weight loss diet (3¾ cup; 908 kcal/day) and a small, unmeasured piece of baked chicken when the first owner prepared his lunch. The owners reported that they had cut back on all other treats but were unable to provide specific quantities. The Spaniel was reported to be moving around better and to now have a waist. The owners were pleased with the progress. At the 5-month phone recheck, the owners reported that the Spaniel was still eating the therapeutic weight loss diet and continued to move around more. The owners did not have an updated weight at the time, but reported that friends are noticing the Spaniel's weight loss. The owners reported that the Spaniel had recently increased water intake and had experienced dorsal hair loss and had scheduled an appointment with the Spaniel's veterinarian for evaluation of these recent changes. Overall, the owners were still pleased with the Spaniel's progress.

The Spaniel's weight loss is an open case. The initial 16-pound lost over the first 4 months was in the target range of 4–8 pounds per month. The nutritionist was very proud of the owners for dramatically altering the Spaniel's management. This case highlights the importance of thorough investigation of diet history and management, and creating a plan that minimizes stress and work for the owners while achieving the weight loss goal.

9.2.5 Discussion

The Spaniel achieved her obese body condition due to an imbalance in energy intake and expenditure, specifically due to excess energy intake. Weight loss will benefit the Spaniel in numerous ways. The Spaniel initially presented to the VTH surgery service for evaluation of lameness. Resolution of obesity will resolve the unnecessary stress on the musculoskeletal system. The owners reported that the Spaniel had improved ambulation within the first 4 months and before ideal body weight was achieved.

The Spaniel's owners successfully implemented a weight loss plan that included careful attention to the current diet and feeding management (i.e., owner lifestyle). Careful consideration of feeding management and daily schedule helps to frame a weight loss plan to minimize stress on the owner. It is the author's experience that improper diet transition can have negative consequences on acceptance of new food, particularly when transitioning away from human food. As an open case, the complete weight loss trajectory is unknown. In the author's experience, some obese patients will plateau in their weight loss. When weight loss plateaus, diet compliance should be evaluated and recommendations should be adjusted. Furthermore, the author's approach to calculating ideal body weight, which influences target daily energy requirements for weight loss, is one approach. Another way to estimate ideal body weight is to subtract the estimated extra 40% body weight from current body weight. At the end of the day, the initial plan is a place to start and the success of the initial plan will be determined through consistent monitoring and reformulation of the diet plan as needed.

KEY LEARNING ISSUES

1. Don't be overwhelmed by the obese dog that has a tremendous amount of body weight to loose.
2. Careful consideration of the current and past diet, and feeding management helps to fine-tune weight loss recommendations.
3. You may need to take time transitioning a morbidly obese dog onto the appropriate diet. Dogs that have been fed a diet largely composed of human food are not likely to take to a weight loss diet quickly.
4. Provide detailed recommendations. Include specific treat recommendations in addition to specific diet recommendations.
5. Recheck, recheck, recheck and remind owners of a job well done.

REFERENCE

1. Brooks D, Churchill J, Fein K et al. 2014 AAHA weight management guidelines for dogs and cats. *Journal of the American Animal Hospital Association* 2014;50(1):1–11.

9.3 CASE 3: ANESTHETIC CONCERNS IN THE OBESE SMALL ANIMAL PATIENT

LYDIA LOVE

9.3.1 Patient history

A 7-year-old female, spayed, domestic shorthair cat presented for general anesthesia for a subtotal colectomy due to primary megacolon and subsequent chronic constipation. The patient had been managed conservatively for 6 months with a therapeutic diet,* lactulose, and compounded cisapride. However, constipation was recurrent and frequent associated hospitalization led the owner to elect surgical intervention.

9.3.2 Patient assessment

The patient weighed 21.8 pounds (9.9 kg) with a BCS of >9/9 (Figure 9.2). Moderate dental disease was noted on physical exam and normal heart and lung sounds were auscultated. Abdominal palpation was difficult due to the obesity but firm stool was felt in the descending colon.

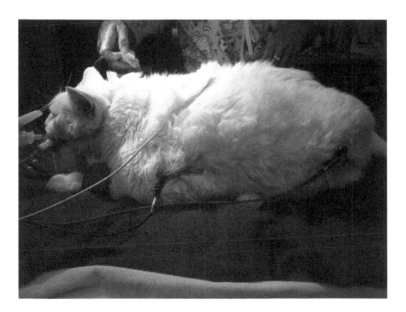

Figure 9.2 An obese, 7-year-old, spayed, female domestic shorthair cat presents for anesthesia.

* Royal Canin Veterinary Diet Gastrointestinal Fiber Response, Royal Canin U.S.A, Inc.

9.3.3 Plan

General anesthesia for a subtotal colectomy was planned. Anesthetic concerns are grouped into patient- and procedure-oriented issues, and for this patient primarily included hypoventilation and hypoxemia, subclinical cardiac dysfunction, correct dosing of sedatives and anesthetics, and management of pain.

The respiratory system of the obese patient is less compliant than normal weight subjects, due to increased fat mass, restrictive breathing patterns, and increased pulmonary blood volume. Inspiratory and expiratory flow limitations may occur and can be accompanied by hypoventilation. Obese patients breathe at low lung volumes and have a decreased functional residual capacity (FRC) relative to those of normal weight. The increased fat mass and small tidal volumes lead to airway closure, subsequent atelectasis, and gas exchange inequalities. Dose-dependent respiratory depression caused by general anesthetics and positioning in dorsal recumbency exacerbate hypoventilation, causing respiratory acidosis and possibly leading to desaturation in the perioperative period. Preoxygenation prior to induction was planned for this obese patient to denitrogenate the FRC and increase oxygen storage in the lungs, extending the time to desaturation (1). During general anesthesia, ventilation was assessed by monitoring end-expiratory carbon dioxide concentrations. Controlled ventilation (manual or mechanical) was used to maintain normal carbon dioxide concentrations, and pulse oximetry was closely followed. Close objective monitoring of oxygenation continued into the recovery period.

Although not as well-described in dogs and cats as it is in humans, the obese patient may display subclinical diastolic cardiac dysfunction, necessitating close monitoring of cardiovascular function during anesthesia and attention to perianesthetic fluid load. Drugs that can cause tachyarrhythmias (especially dissociative anesthetics and anticholinergics) are avoided, as faster heart rates may limit cardiac filling when diastolic dysfunction is present. Intravenous crystalloid infusion is calculated at surgical rates but based on ideal body weight. Total fluid load is kept under 10–15 mL/kg in the immediate perioperative time period, barring major intraoperative blood loss.

Dose reductions of sedatives and anesthetics are calculated due to obesity-associated changes in pharmacokinetic parameters. As total body weight increases due to increasing fat weight, lean body weight also increases but not in parallel. Most anesthetics and sedatives are moderately to highly lipophilic, which promotes their movement across the blood–brain barrier to their site of action. Therefore, dosing on total body weight (TBW) in the obese patient may lead to a relative overdose. However, ideal body weight (IBW)–based calculations may underdose the patient and a universal dosing scalar has not been established in obese cats and dogs. Drug calculations for this patient were based on adjusted body weight (ABW) (IBW + 0.4 [TBW − IBW]) to account for increased lean body weight (2). However, all anesthetics drugs were titrated to effect while monitoring for cardiorespiratory side effects.

A subtotal colectomy is an invasive abdominal procedure that requires dorsal recumbency for a moderate length of time (typically less than 2 hours). In addition to the aforementioned increase in atelectasis and hypoventilation, dorsal recumbency in the obese patient could aggravate joint disease and possibly lead to pressure-related nerve and muscle complications. Extra padding was placed on the surgical table and the cat's limbs were placed in a comfortable position. Finally, moderate to severe pain is expected in the immediate postoperative period following abdominal surgery and a multimodal preventative analgesic plan was employed in the perioperative time period.

9.3.4 Short- and long-term follow-up

The patient was >40% overweight and IBW was estimated at 13.5 pounds (6.1 kg) (3). Ideal body weight was estimated because suggested methodology for calculating IBW* has not been validated in patients who are severely obese (BCS >9/9) (3). All drugs doses were calculated based on ABW (16.8 pounds [7.6 kg]).

The patient was premedicated with fentanyl (5 mcg/kg) intravenously and a transflectance pulse oximeter probe was attached to the shaved base of the tail. An oscillometric noninvasive arterial blood pressure cuff and ECG leads were attached. A tight-fitting facemask was used to preoxygenate the patient for 5 minutes and she was then induced to anesthesia with a combination of ketamine (2 mg/kg) and propofol (1.8 mg/kg). Coinduction with ketamine allows reduction of propofol requirements and results in a better hemodynamic profile at induction (4). Anesthesia was maintained with a partial intravenous technique including sevoflurane in 100% oxygen titrated to effect with fentanyl (10 mcg/kg/hr) and ketamine (0.6 mg/kg/hr) infusions. An epidural was considered, but the anatomical landmarks were difficult to palpate.

In the operating room, the patient was placed in dorsal recumbency and mechanical ventilation with a time-cycled, volume-controlled, pressure-limited anesthesia ventilator was initiated. A 5 cmH$_2$O positive end-expiratory pressure (PEEP) valve was placed in the expiratory limb of the breathing circuit. Monitoring included continuous pulse oximetry, noninvasive oscillometric blood pressure, capnography, temperature, and lead II electrocardiography. Minor hypotension was treated by reducing the inhalant and administering one bolus of ephedrine (0.03 mg/kg) intravenously. The patient's temperature remained above 100°F throughout without active external warming.

At the end of the procedure, inhalant anesthesia was discontinued and the fentanyl and ketamine infusions were reduced by 50%. The patient was turned to lateral recumbency and allowed to breathe 100% oxygen spontaneously. During spontaneous ventilation, end tidal carbon dioxide concentrations were upward of 55 mm Hg. In order to avoid hypoxemia from hypoventilation, a nasal oxygen line was placed to continue oxygen supplementation in the recovery period (Figure 9.3). Oxygen was supplemented at 50 mL/kg/min until the next morning. The pulse oximetry transflectance probe was maintained at the tail base for continued oxygen saturation monitoring. Analgesic infusions were tapered over the first 12 hours of

* IBW = (Current BW × [100 – %Body fat])/0.8.

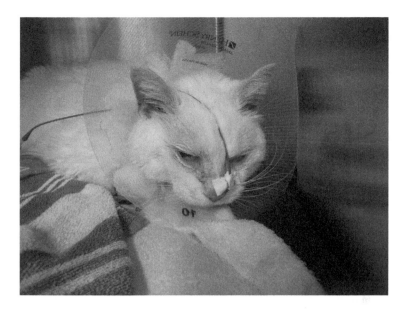

Figure 9.3 The obese patient in the anesthesia recovery unit with a nasal line in place to supplement inspired oxygen and decrease the risk of hypoxemia due to residual hypoventilation and atelectasis.

recovery and de-escalation of analgesic coverage was accomplished by administering long-acting buprenorphine (0.27 mg/kg SQ)* the next morning. Long-acting buprenorphine was repeated 24 hours later prior to discharge, 37 hours after recovery from anesthesia.

9.3.5 Discussion

Increasing body mass index in humans is associated with longer anesthetic times, longer surgical times, increased risk of respiratory and renal complications, increased risk of infection, longer hospital stays, and increased cost in the perioperative time period (5,6). It is likely that many of these issues are relevant to obese, small animal anesthetic patients as well and the increased use of resources should be anticipated.

The risks of anesthesia are mitigated by anticipating possible complications, constructing strategies to circumvent those complications, monitoring for development of expected and unexpected complications, and being prepared to respond to perianesthetic issues as they arise. In obese patients the primary concerns surround respiratory function and dose reductions of anesthetic and sedative agents.

Preoxygenation is advised in all patients prior to induction of anesthesia to avoid desaturation. Because obese patients have increased metabolic demands coupled with a much smaller FRC, desaturation can occur rapidly at induction.

* Simbadol, Zoetis, Inc.

The patient of this report was preoxygenated for 5 minutes and then rapidly intubated and ventilated by hand. During the maintenance phase, the patient was placed on a mechanical ventilator. There is no consensus on perianesthetic ventilation strategies in obese human patients and no published information regarding this topic in cats and dogs. Tidal volumes are probably best based on IBW to avoid baro- or volutrauma. An alveolar recruitment maneuver with the addition of PEEP reduces atelectasis and improves compliance and gas exchange in obese human patients during anesthesia (7). A PEEP valve was utilized during anesthesia in the patient of this case report, but an alveolar recruitment maneuver was not performed as no episodes of hypoxemia were noted. After discontinuing mechanical ventilation, but while still being supplemented with 100% oxygen, hypoventilation was documented. To avoid desaturation due to continued hypoventilation and ventilation–perfusion mismatch caused by residual atelectasis, a nasal oxygen line was placed and the patient was monitored objectively with continuous pulse oximetry throughout recovery.

Finally, initial drug doses were calculated for this patient based on an ABW. Not enough information is available even for humans to make firm recommendations about drug dosing in obesity and very few pharmacokinetic–pharmacodynamic studies have been conducted in obese subjects of any species. Ideally, species- and drug-specific guidelines would exist, but lacking those, using ideal body weight plus a percentage of excess weight may account for the nonlinear increase in lean body weight that occurs as TBW increases. More generally, anesthetic agents are best titrated carefully to effect while monitoring for cardiorespiratory side effects.

KEY LEARNING ISSUES

Safety in anesthesia, for obese as well as normal weight subjects, is dictated not by a certain drug or drug combination but by good monitoring and supportive care.

1. Hypoventilation and hypoxemia are among the most common perianesthetic complications for obese cats and dogs, and the respiratory system should be monitored closely.
2. Lacking specific pharmacokinetic–pharmacodynamic information, anesthetic and sedative drug doses should be calculated on adjusted body weight and then titrated to effect.

REFERENCES

1. McNally EM, Robertson SA, Pablo LS. Comparison of time to desaturation between preoxygenated and nonpreoxygenated dogs following sedation with acepromazine maleate and morphine and induction of anesthesia with propofol. *American Journal of Veterinary Research* 2009 November;70(11):1333–1338.

2. Servin F, Farinotti R, Haberer JP et al. Propofol infusion for maintenance of anesthesia in morbidly obese patients receiving nitrous oxide a clinical and pharmacokinetic study. *Anesthesiology* 1993 April;78(4):657–665.
3. Brooks B, Churchill J, Fein K et al. 2014 AAHA weight management guidelines for dogs and cats. *Journal of the American Animal Hospital Association* 2014 January–February;50(1):1–11.
4. Martinez-Taboada F, Leece EA. Comparison of propofol with ketofol, a propofol-ketamine admixture, for induction of anaesthesia in healthy dogs. *Veterinary Anaesthesia and Analgesia* 2014 November;41(6): 575–582.
5. Higgins DM, Mallory GW, Planchard R et al. Understanding the impact of obesity on short-term outcomes and in-hospital costs after instrumented spinal fusion. *Neurosurgery* 2016 January;78(1):127–132.
6. Ranum D, Ma H, Shapiro FE et al. Analysis of patient injury based on anesthesiology closed claims data from a major malpractice insurer. *Journal of Healthcare Risk Managemant* 2014;34(2):31–42.
7. Aldenkortt M, Lysakowski C, Elia N et al. Ventilation strategies in obese patients undergoing surgery: A quantitative systematic review and meta-analysis. *British Journal of Anaesthsia* 2012 October;109(4):493–502.

9.4 CASE 4: ESTIMATING DEGREE OF OBESITY FOR WEIGHT LOSS PLANNING IN AN OBESE DOMESTIC SHORTHAIR CAT

CHARLOTTE REINHARD BJØRNVAD

9.4.1 Patient history

A 6.5-year-old male, castrated, indoor confined domestic shorthair (DSH) presented to the clinical nutrition service at a veterinary teaching hospital after referral from a private practice that had seen the cat for a dental cleaning. Following the dental cleaning, the cat was referred to the service because it was diagnosed as obese and the owner was committed to trying a weight loss plan. The owner informed the clinician that the cat was sedentary and there were no other pets in the household. The cat was fed an indoor cat maintenance dry diet *ad libitum* and given a little bit of milk, some cheese snacks, and chicken or tuna a couple of times a day; the owner did not know the exact quantities. Hematology and biochemistry from the referring veterinarian showed normal values except for a hypercholesterolemia 7.54 mmol/L (reference 2.46–3.37 mmol/L) following an overnight fast.

9.4.2 Patient assessment

During the physical examination, the cat had normal vital signs, and no abnormalities were identified apart from excessive fat covering the ribs, no discernible waist, and a marked inguinal fat pad. Body weight (BW) was 10.8 kg and body condition score (BCS) was determined to be 9/9 (1). The patient's problem list included obesity and hypercholesterolemia.

9.4.3 Plan

A weight loss plan was calculated based on the 2014 American Animal Hospital Association (AAHA) weight management guidelines for dogs and cats (2). BCS 9/9 was estimated to equal 45% body fat. Based on this, ideal BW was calculated. Calculation of ideal BW:

$$10.8 \text{ kg} \times (100\% - 45\%)/0.8 = 7.4 \text{ kg}$$

With a severely overweight cat, it is important to introduce a slow weight loss plan to reduce the risk of the cat developing hepatic lipidosis (3). The cat should be monitored closely and the owner instructed in reacting if the cat stops eating.

Daily energy requirement was estimated to be 80% of RER for an expected weight loss of 0.5%–2% per week, which is generally considered a safe weight loss rate (2):

Calculation of resting energy requirement (RER):

$$70 \times (\text{Ideal BW})^{0.75} = 70 \times 7.4^{0.75} = 314 \text{ kcal/day}$$

Calculation of daily energy allocation for weight loss:

$$0.8 \times 314 = 251 \text{ kcal/day}$$

Energy distribution of the commercial weight loss diet chosen:

Nutrient	As fed	ME
Protein (%)	34	42
Fat (%)	9	24
Carbohydrate (%)	28	34
Metabolizable energy (ME) (kcal/kg)	3090	

Calculation of amount to feed:

$$251/3090 \times 1000 \text{ g/kg} = 81 \text{ grams/day (divided in two equal portions)}$$

National Research Council (NRC) recommended allowance of protein for cats (4):

$$4.96 \text{ g protein} \times (\text{Ideal BW})^{0.67} = 4.96 \times 7.4^{0.67} = 19 \text{ g/day}$$

Calculation of protein level with advised feeding:

$$0.34 \times 81 \text{ g} = 27.5 \text{ g/day}$$

The owner was informed to feed only the recommended diet and if she wanted to give snacks to save some of the allocated ration for this.

9.4.4 Short-term follow-up

The cat presented for a recheck after 14 days. Expected weight loss was approximately 200 grams. However, the cat had only lost 20 grams. The owner informed that she had been following the prescription and only fed the advocated amount strictly for all 2 weeks, despite that the cat was begging for treats. The cat did not have access to food from elsewhere. Because we had just started recruiting for a clinical weight loss trial, the owner was asked if she would like her cat to be included. She accepted and the cat was entered in the trial. At inclusion, blood samples and urine were analyzed and no abnormalities were identified on complete blood count, serum biochemistry (except for a fasted hypercholesterolemia 8.66 mmol/L [reference 2.46–3.37 mmol/L]), total thyroxine (T4), or urinalysis. Subsequently the body composition was determined using dual energy x-ray absorptiometry (DEXA; Figure 9.4) and using this methodology, body fat percentage (BF%) was determined to be 60.2%. Based on the new measurement, a new weight loss plan was calculated according to the AAHA weight loss guidelines (2).

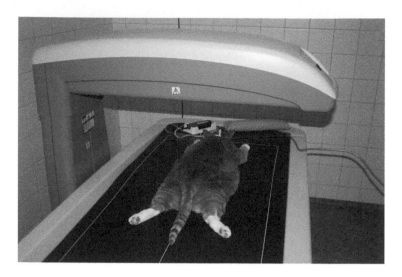

Figure 9.4 Cat being scanned in a dual energy x-ray absorptiometry scanner. (Photo by K.M. Hoelmkjaer.)

Calculation of ideal BW for a BF% of 60%:

$$\text{Current BW} \times (100 - \%BF)/0.8 = 10.8 \times (100\% - 60\%)/0.8 = 5.4\,kg$$

Calculation of resting energy requirement (RER):

$$70 \times 5.4^{0.75} = 248\,kcal/day$$

Calculation of daily energy allocation for weight loss:

$$0.8 \times 248\,kcal = 198\,kcal/day$$

The cat liked the prescribed weight loss diet and it was decided to continue feeding this diet:
Calculation of amount to feed:

$$198/3090 \times 1000\,g/kg = 64\,grams/day\,(divided\ in\ two\ equal\ portions)$$

NRC recommended allowance of protein for cats:

$$4.96\,g\ protein \times (\text{Ideal BW})^{0.67} = 4.96 \times 5.4^{0.67} = 15.4\,g/day$$

Calculation of protein level with advised feeding:

$$0.34 \times 64\,g/day = 21.8\,g/day$$

9.4.5 Discussion

Based on the actual body fat percentage (BF%), it was discovered that during the last 14 days, the cat had been fed what equaled its RER for its ideal BW and had not been restricted to a level where weight loss could be anticipated. After adjustment to a BF% of 60%, the cat started to lose weight at the rate of 1% per week. The BCS system is good for determining if an animal is underweight, lean, or obese, but care should be taken when estimating the degree of fatness (BF%) based on a BCS. BF% relating to a BCS may depend on age, breed, and lifestyle, and may therefore differ between individuals both in cats and dogs (1,5,6). This case underscores the particular problem of assessing the BF% of an animal whose fatness exceeds the BCS scale (score 9/9 equals 45% body fat) and it highlights the limitations of using the 9-point body condition score for extremely overweight animals. To increase the accuracy in determining energy restriction for a particular individual, there are different complementary methods that should be added whenever possible. If DEXA scanning is not an option, the examination of animals with a BCS of 7–9/9 should be supplemented with the feline Body Fat Index (BFI) scoring system (7). The feline BFI was designed to determine higher BF%s than the BCS with a limit at 65% body fat (BFI 70). It is a relatively new method and has only been validated once, thus its usefulness in improving BF% estimates is not certain, but it could serve as a valuable complementary method for obese patients. In addition, if at all possible, calculating the energy allocation given to the cat before initiation of a weight loss plan could support the estimation of RER and required energy restriction. In the beginning of a weight loss plan, frequent rechecks are necessary, as they enable you to detect if weight loss is not achieved on current recommendations and it stimulates owner compliance. Some cats may become very stressed by the frequent visits to the veterinarian. For those, it is possible to manage some rechecks long distance, that is, the owner weighs the cat at home followed by a telephone consultation. Also, take into account that lack of results could have many explanations including incorrect estimation of ideal BW, lack of owner compliance, and access to food elsewhere, or a combination of these. Thus, be sure to thoroughly investigate causes for lacking results.

KEY LEARNING ISSUES

1. For animals with a BCS of 8–9/9 supplement the examination with the BFI that is designed to determine higher BF% and if possible calculations of current daily energy intake.
2. Frequent rechecks to detect if weight loss is not achieved on current recommendations.
3. Take into account that lack of results could have many explanations including incorrect estimation of ideal BW, lack of owner compliance, and access to food elsewhere.

REFERENCES

1. Laflamme D. Development and validation of a body condition score system for cats: A clinical tool. *Feline Practice* 1997;25(5/6):13–18.
2. Brooks D, Churchill J, Fein K et al. 2014 AAHA weight management guidelines for dogs and cats. *Journal of the American Animal Hospital Association* 2014;50(1):1–11.
3. Armstrong PJ, Blanchard G. Hepatic lipidosis in cats. *Veterinary Clinics Small Animals* 2009;39:599–616.
4. National Research Council of the National Academies. Nutrient requirements and dietary nutrient concentrations. In: *Nutrient Requirements of Dogs and Cats*. Washington, DC: National Academies Press; 2006, pp. 354–370.
5. Bjornvad CR, Nielsen DH, Armstrong PJ et al. Evaluation of a nine-point body condition scoring system in physically inactive pet cats. *American Journal of Veterinary Research* 2011;72(4):433–437.
6. Jeusette I, Greco D, Aquino F et al. Effect of breed on body composition and comparison between various methods to estimate body composition in dogs. *Research in Veterinary Science* 2010;88(2):227–232.
7. Witzel AL, Kirk CA, Henry GA, Toll PW, Brejda JJ, Paetau-Robinson I. Use of a morphometric method and body fat index system for estimation of body composition in overweight and obese cats. *Journal of the American Veterinary Medical Association* 2014;244(11):1285–1290.

9.5 CASE 5: REMISSION OF DIABETES MELLITUS FOLLOWING WEIGHT LOSS IN A DOMESTIC SHORTHAIR CAT

ANDREW MCGLINCHEY AND MARTHA G. CLINE

9.5.1 Patient history

A 13-year-old spayed, female, domestic shorthair cat was presented to the clinical nutrition service at a specialty hospital after her primary care veterinarian referred her for nutritional management of diabetes mellitus (DM) and obesity. She had been diagnosed with DM 4 months prior to presentation after evaluation of polyuria and polydipsia (PU/PD). Blood work at that time revealed mild hyperalbuminemia (4.1 g/dL, reference range 2.5–3.9), hyperglycemia (412 mg/dL, reference range 64–170), and hypertriglyceridemia (304 mg/dL, reference range 25–160), with the remainder of parameters within normal limits. Urinalysis revealed glucosuria and no ketonuria. At presentation to the nutrition service, she was on insulin glargine (100 U/mL)* at 2 units every 12 hours. Her owners noted negative ketonuria and positive glucosuria when repeatedly measured at home. A subsequent fructosamine measurement 3 months after diagnosis was consistent with good control of her DM (350 μmol/L, reference range 142–450). A blood glucose curve had not been performed due to patient temperament. Her PU/PD had resolved at that time and her body weight was stable.

9.5.2 Patient assessment

At the time of presentation, the patient was fed 1/4 cup (8 oz measuring cup) of a therapeutic extruded diet,†,‡ marketed for diabetic patients and approximately 1 teaspoon of the canned version of the same diet in the morning and at night. She was also given one treat marketed for joint health twice per day.§ Her total calorie consumption at the time was estimated to be approximately 319 kcal per day.

Initial physical examination revealed moderate dental calculi, gingival hyperemia, and obesity. Her body weight (BW) was 8.1 kg, with a body condition score (BCS) of 9/9 (1), an estimated body fat of 50%, and good muscle condition. The remainder of her general physical examination revealed no significant findings. Her significant problem list at that time included DM, obesity, and periodontal disease.

---

* Lantus Insulin, Sanofi.

† Purina ProPlan Veterinary Diets DM Dietetic Management® Feline Formula dry (592 kcal/cup, 4118 kcal/kg, protein 50% ME, fat 37% ME, carbohydrate 13% ME).

‡ Purina ProPlan Veterinary Diets DM Dietetic Management® Feline Formula canned (191 kcal/can, 1227 kcal/kg, protein 38.8% ME, fat 58% ME, carbohydrate 3.3% ME).

§ GNC Ultra Mega Hip and Joint Health treats (5.4 kcal per treat).

9.5.3 Plan

A weight loss plan was recommended to address the patient's obesity and to improve insulin sensitivity. Based on her initial BW and estimated body fat of 50%, it was estimated that her ideal BW was approximately 5.4 kg.

$$\text{Calculation of ideal BW} = \text{Current body weight}$$
$$\times [(100 - \text{Current body fat\%})/(100 - \text{Ideal body fat\%})]$$
$$8.1 \text{ kg} \times (100\% - 50\%)/(100\% - 25\%) = 5.4 \text{ kg}$$

Due to the patient's advanced age and evidence to suggest that female cats have a higher body fat percentage at a body condition score of 5/9 (3), an ideal body fat percentage of 25% was selected for this patient. A body fat percentage of 20%–24% has been recommended to correlate with a BCS of 5/9 in both dogs and cats (2).

Resting energy requirement (RER) for her ideal body weight was calculated at 250 kcal/day:

$$\text{Calculation of RER} = (\text{Body weight kg})^{0.75} \times 70$$
$$5.4 \text{ kg}^{7.5} \times 70 = 248 \text{ kcal/day}$$

In order to safely attain her weight loss goal at a rate of 0.5%–2% BW per week (2), her maintenance energy requirement (MER) was calculated using a life stage factor of 0.8.

$$\text{Calculation of MER} = \text{Life stage factor} \times \text{RER}$$
$$0.8 \times 248 = 198 \text{ kcal/day}$$

The client was instructed to feed the previously recommended diet in one of two combinations approximating her caloric requirements (see Table 9.2), with the prescribed insulin administered 30 minutes following each meal. The treat marketed for joint health was also incorporated into the diet plan, with 1 given every 12 hours.

The owner was instructed to monitor daily for glucosuria and watch for signs of hypoglycemia due to the potential for improved insulin sensitivity with weight loss. It was recommended to follow-up in 2 weeks to ensure a safe and effective rate of weight loss. It was also recommended to reassess diabetic control in 2 weeks with a serum fructosamine measurement as the patient's temperament did not allow for a blood glucose curve in hospital or at home.

Table 9.2 The owner's were given two feeding options: (1) ½ can every 12 hours or (2) 1/3 can and 8 grams of dry every 12 hours

Daily amount	kcal/day from canned	kcal/day from dry	kcal/day from treats	Total kcal/day
Option 1	191	0	10.8	201.8
Option 2	127	66	10.8	203.8

9.5.4 Short- and long-term follow-up

The patient rechecked with her regular veterinarian approximately 2 weeks after starting her weight loss plan. Her body weight was 7.9 kg with a rate of weight loss of 1.2% per week. Approximately 4 weeks after starting her weight loss plan, the patient presented to her regular veterinarian due to repeated negative glucosuria at home. Blood glucose measurement at the time was 98 mg/dL (reference range 64–170). Her body weight was 7.7 kg indicating an acceptable rate of weight loss at 1.2% of BW per week with a total weight loss of 0.4 kg or 4.9% of her body weight. Insulin was discontinued due to suspected remission. No changes were made to her weight loss plan at the time and her owners were instructed to continue to monitor for glucosuria following discontinuation of her insulin.

The patient's weight was rechecked every 4 weeks. The MER was recalculated and amount fed was adjusted as necessary to maintain an acceptable rate of weight loss. Fifteen months after initiation of the weight loss program, the patient had reached her target BW of 5.4 kg, for a total loss of 2.7 kg or 31% BW. She remained in diabetic remission the length of her weight loss plan.

9.5.5 Discussion

Diabetes mellitus (DM) in cats occurs commonly due to peripheral insulin resistance as a result of excess adiposity and beta cell dysfunction (4). Cats can have insulin resistance at just 10% over their lean body weight (5). Obese cats are up to 3.9 times as likely to have DM than cats with an ideal BCS (6). Every 1 kg increase in body weight has been associated with a 30% decrease in insulin sensitivity, which was normalized with weight loss (7). Weight loss should be a primary goal in overweight/obese cats with DM to help achieve and maintain diabetic remission in conjunction with appropriate medical management. The timing of weight management should be delayed in an overtly ill cat until stabilized.

A survey of veterinarians in the Southeastern United States revealed that 97% (87/90) of vets always or usually recommended dietary management at the time of DM diagnosis and 93% of respondents recommended diets marked as low carbohydrate (LC) (8). The number of veterinarians recommending weight loss was not determined in this study. A diet with a carbohydrate content of approximately 35 g/1000 kcal or less (9,13) may be advantageous for cats with DM. Cats fed a LC–low fiber diet appeared to be better regulated and had a significantly higher remission rate of 68% compared to cats fed a moderate carbohydrate–high fiber diet with a remission rate of 41% (10). It is notable that postprandial hyperglycemia, which causes further beta-cell toxicity and exacerbates DM, is increased in magnitude and duration in some overweight cats (11). Therefore, correction of obesity is important to achieve and maintain diabetic remission, as seen in the described patient. Switching to a LC diet alone without addressing the patient's excess body weight did not result in remission of this patient's DM.

The authors typically recommend a canned, LC therapeutic weight loss diet for cats with DM due to the higher moisture content, lower calorie density, and ease of portion control when compared to dry LC diets. A dry food may be preferred by some patients and cat owners. A low calorie density, high protein (≥115 g/1000 kcal) weight loss diet may be recommended in these cases to improve owner and patient compliance with higher feeding volumes when compared to LC, high calorie density dry diets. These dry diets may be lower in fat and/or have supplemental fiber to reduce calorie density. Diets containing high amounts of protein (≥115 g/1000 kcal) are recommended to support lean body mass during a weight loss plan for a diabetic patient. Specific feeding amounts during weight loss should be recommended and *ad libitum* feeding of dry food is not recommended. The authors recommend weighing dry food on a kitchen gram scale for improved accuracy when feeding (12). This can be calculated using the caloric information (kcal/kg) provided on the pet food label.

KEY LEARNING ISSUES

1. This patient's diabetes mellitus did not achieve remission with appropriate medical management and a low carbohydrate diet until weight loss was initiated. Weight loss is essential in overweight/obese cats to improve peripheral insulin sensitivity.
2. Veterinarians and pet owners should recognize and address obesity in diabetic feline patients at the time of diagnosis once the patient is stabilized and throughout treatment.
3. Client education on overweight/obesity's impact on diabetic control is as important as making general diet recommendations.
4. High protein diets that are low carbohydrate or fiber supplemented may be used as part of a weight loss plan in diabetic feline patients. There is evidence that feeding a low carbohydrate, high protein diet may be advantageous in reducing the insulin requirement in cats, but specific diet recommendations should be tailored to the individual patient.

REFERENCES

1. Laflamme D. Development and validation of a body condition score system for cats: A clinical tool. *Feline Practice* 1997;25:13–17.
2. Brooks D, Churchill J, Fein K, Linder D, Michel KE, Tudor K, Ward E, Witzel A. 2014 AAHA weight management guidelines for dogs and cats. *Journal of the American Animal Hospital Association* 2014;50:1–11.
3. Bjornvad CR, Nielsen DH, Armstrong PJ, McEvoy F, Hoelmkjaer KM, Jensen KS, Pedersen GF, Kristensen AT. Evaluation of a nine-point body condition scoring system in physically inactive pet cats. *American Journal of Veterinary Research* 2011;72:433–437.
4. Rand JS, Fleeman LM, Farrow HA, Appleton DJ, Lederer R. Canine and feline diabetes mellitus: Nature or nurture? *Journal of Nutrition* 2004;134:2072S–2080S.

5. Hoenig M, Pach N, Thomaseth K, Le A, Schaeffer D, Ferguson DC. Cats differ from other species in their cytokine and antioxidant enzyme response when developing obesity. *Obesity (Silver Spring)* 2003;21:E407–E414.

6. Scarlett JM, Donoghue S. Associations between body condition and disease in cats. *Journal of the American Veterinary Medical Association* 1998;212:1725–1731.

7. Hoenig M, Thomaseth K, Waldron M, Ferguson DC. Insulin sensitivity, fat distribution, and adipocytokine response to different diets in lean and obese cats before and after weight loss. *American Journal of Physiology: Regulatory, Integrative and Comparative Physiology* 2007;292:R227–R234.

8. Smith JR, Vrono Z, Rapoport GS, Turek MM, Creevy KE. A survey of Southeastern United States veterinarians' preferences for managing cats with diabetes mellitus. *Journal of Feline Medicine and Surgery* 2012;14:716–722.

9. Behrend E, Holford A, Lathan P, Rucinsky R, Schulman R. 2018 AAHA diabetes management guidelines for dogs and cats. *Journal of the American Animal Hospital Association* 2018;54:1–21.

10. Bennett N, Greco DS, Peterson ME, Kirk C, Mathes M, Fettman MJ. Comparison of a low carbohydrate-low fiber diet and a moderate carbohydrate-high fiber diet in the management of feline diabetes mellitus. *Journal of Feline Medicine and Surgery* 2006;8:73–84.

11. Coradini M, Rand JS, Morton JM, Rawlings JM. Effects of two commercially available feline diets on glucose and insulin concentrations, insulin sensitivity and energetic efficiency of weight gain. *British Journal of Nutrition* 2011;106(Suppl 1):S64–S77.

12. German AJ, Holden SL, Mason SL, Bryner C, Bouldoires C, Morris PJ, Deboise M, Biourge V. Imprecision when using measuring cups to weigh out extruded dry kibbled food. *Journal of Animal Physiology and Animal Nutrition* 2011;95:368–373.

13. Bonagura JD, Twedt DC. *Kirk's Current Veterinary Therapy (CVT) XIV*. 14th ed. Elsevier, St. Louis, MO 2008:201.

9.6 CASE 6: BEHAVIORAL MANAGEMENT OF OBESITY

DEBORAH E. LINDER AND MEGAN K. MUELLER

9.6.1 Patient history

Jacob presented as an overweight, 2-year-old, neutered, male Labrador retriever for a weight management consultation after a recent diagnosis of an anterior cruciate ligament tear and surgical correction with a lateral suture repair. An initial diet history revealed that he was receiving 600 kcal/d from an over-the-counter weight management dry dog food and additional unknown calories from table scraps with each meal, which varied daily depending on what the family had for dinner. Cheese and deli meat were used to administer an anti-inflammatory medication twice daily, which added an additional 100 kcal/d.

9.6.2 Patient assessment

Jacob was 44 kg (97 lb) on presentation with a BCS of 8/9 and normal muscle condition. Other than mild to moderate pain on limb extension, a physical examination and screening laboratory work (including a complete blood count, chemistry panel, urinalysis, and thyroid level) did not reveal significant abnormalities, and his ideal weight was estimated to be 34 kg (74 lb). This ideal weight was determined by referencing a previous weight in the medical record when Jacob was determined an ideal 5/9 body condition score (1).

9.6.3 Plan

Jacob was initially placed on exercise restriction for 8 weeks after the surgical procedure. During this time, his weight management plan consisted solely of dietary management. The family was switched to a therapeutic weight loss food given Jacob's need for caloric restriction and lack of exercise. Initial calorie intake was set at resting energy requirements for ideal weight (1) of 34 kg (this was calculated with the formula: $70 \times [\text{Body weight in kg}]^{0.75} = 70 \times 34^{0.75} =$ approximately 1000 kcal/day).

A daily feeding schedule was discussed for Jacob that included 1000 kcal total with 900 kcal in a therapeutic weight loss food and 10% of the total 1000 kcal (100 kcal) reserved for Jacob's favorite treats.

9.6.4 Short- and long-term follow-up

Jacob was weighed weekly and his food intake was adjusted to meet a goal rate of weight loss (0.5%–1% of weight loss per week) (1). While discussing the plan with the owner at the 2-week check-in, there was significant concern that Jacob was restless, acting out by trying to get into trash and destroying the owners' clothing, and only got excited at meal time, which lasted only 10 seconds according to the owner. Even though he was receiving a larger volume of food on the therapeutic diet, he ate his food quickly and enthusiastically, but then went back to being restless until the next meal. On further discussion, the owner also felt guilty over not allowing Jacob to go on walks or play in the pond near their house. He did not want his dog to resent him or their time together. The owner felt that the meals were the only enjoyable part of his dog's daily routine and hated that it was over so quickly, so he wanted to provide more meals and treats until Jacob could exercise more.

It was discussed with the owner that the exercise restriction was necessary for proper recovery and that adding food or treats would add weight and make Jacob feel even worse, as overweight pets have more pain and emotional disturbance (2). Options were discussed as highlighted in the American Animal Hospital Association (AAHA) 2014 weight management guidelines troubleshooting tips for behavioral management (1), including using food-dispensing toys and food puzzles that would prolong mealtime. The owner really liked the idea of making mealtime into a game that would extend Jacob's enjoyment and allow the owner to experience quality time with the pet as well. For one meal a day, the owner used pieces of the kibble to teach Jacob new tricks that prolonged feeding. For example, the owner taught him to stay while he placed one piece of kibble on each of his paws and to wait before eating each, as seen in Figure 9.5. This resolved the

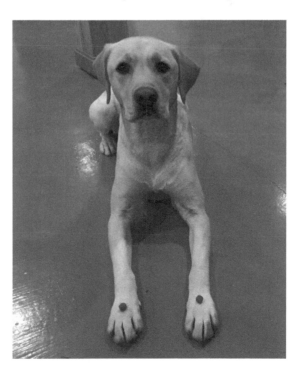

Figure 9.5 For one meal a day, the owner used pieces of the kibble to teach Jacob new tricks that prolonged feeding. In this photo, the owner taught him to stay while he placed one piece of kibble on each of his paws and to wait before eating each.

owner's concern, and at their 8-week recheck, Jacob was 35 kg (77 lb), and the family was continuing to follow the agreed-on plan.

9.6.5 Discussion

Seeing Jacob show enthusiasm and enjoy their time together was an important aspect of the relationship between the owner and Jacob. For both the owner and Jacob to benefit from positive interaction, Jacob's food motivation was encouraged as a time to explore creative ways to interact incorporating mental stimulation and game playing into mealtime. Instead of allowing Jacob to eat all his food quickly, the owner engaged the dog in positive training that allowed them to strengthen their bond without negatively affecting the weight management plan. The owner was able to see Jacob enjoy learning new tricks and excitedly finding parts of his meal as he spent time with the owner.

KEY LEARNING ISSUES

1. Obesity is a complex nutritional disorder that often requires comprehensive management beyond a standard diet and exercise program to be successful.
2. Effective client communication can assist the veterinary team in appreciating each family's unique relationship with the pets in the household and keep the human–animal bond intact.
3. Obesity treatment can be multimodal and include management from both medical and psychological perspectives to achieve success in behavioral management.
4. Weight management plans can be created together with veterinarians and pet owners in a way that reinforces owners' relationship with their pets and does not threaten their bond.

REFERENCES

1. Brooks D, Churchill J, Fein K, Linder D, Michel KE, Tudor K, Ward E, Witzel A. 2014 AAHA weight management guidelines for dogs and cats. *Journal of the American Animal Hospital Association* 2014;50:1–11.
2. German AJ, Holden SL, Wiseman-Orr ML, Reid J, Nolan AM, Biourge V, Morris PJ, Scott EM. Quality of life is reduced in obese dogs but improves after successful weight loss. *Veterinary Journal* 2012;19:428–434.

9.7 CASE 7: CALORIC RESTRICTION, EXERCISE, AND THERAPEUTIC WEIGHT LOSS DURING A NOVEL PROTEIN DIET TRIAL

JUSTIN SHMALBERG

9.7.1 Patient history

A 2-year-old, neutered, male, mixed, large breed dog was presented to a board certified dermatologist for evaluation of nonseasonal pruritus observed since 3 months of age. The owner reported diffuse pruritus, and historical dermatologic lesions were intermittent and developed first on the paws with eventual spread to the ventrum, inguinal, axillary, and aural regions. Secondary bacterial and *Malassezia* infections were common. Serum IgE antibodies were detected against multiple trees, grasses, weeds, molds, insects, and indoor allergens. Antibodies to dietary antigens were also reported; these included eggs, oats, potatoes, rice, and soy. The patient's previous management included recurrent cephalexin administration, ketoconazole, hydroxyzine, numerous empiric maintenance diet trials based on serum IgE testing, immunotherapy injections, and intermittent tapering doses of glucocorticoid. A partial response was observed with either antifungal or antibiotic therapy, and the 18-month immunotherapy protocol had not ameliorated clinical signs. The patient had progressively gained weight and the owner reported this occurred after skeletal maturity.

9.7.2 Patient assessment

The patient was obese with a body condition score (BCS) of 9/9, a body weight of 62.7 kg, and normal musculature (muscle condition score of 3/3). The patient's vital signs were within normal limits, and cardiothoracic auscultation was unremarkable. The dog was diffusely pruritic with ventral abdominal pustules, papules, and epidermal collarettes. Mild erythema was noted in the interdigital spaces of all four paws. Bilateral epidermal crusts and multifocal truncal alopecia were present. He resisted coxofemoral extension on the right hind limb and displayed decreased range of motion at that joint. No other abnormal findings were identified.

The patient's dermatologic lesions were consistent with secondary bacterial pyoderma and Malassezia pododermatitis. Differential diagnoses for the inciting cause included atopic dermatitis, flea allergy dermatitis, contact allergy, or food hypersensitivity. The dermatologist prescribed trimethoprim–sulfadiazine (TMS), topical triamcinolone, ketoconazole, and a medicated shampoo. Nutritional consultation was advised for assessment of the current dietary intake, the potential for a food elimination trial, and to achieve weight loss. The client was feeding a commercially available rabbit-based grain-free dry kibble,* which provided an

* Nature's Variety Instinct Rabbit Meal Formula, 482 kcal/cup, 3988 kcal/kg.

estimated daily caloric intake of 1928 kcal. Dried duck treats* were offered, with an average reported consumption of three treats daily (57 kcal). No supplemental foods were reported. The patient's previous exposure history included a number of commercial foods, and the patient's diet was switched every 2–3 months to evaluate response. A survey of the products revealed that the patient had also consumed beef, bison, lamb, venison, whitefish, egg, tuna, and an equally broad assortment of vegetables and grains. The referring veterinarian selected the rabbit diet as a novel protein diet trial on the basis of its inclusion on a list provided following IgE testing and because the promotional materials indicated that the diet "may provide relief from most food allergy symptoms." However, the diet contained salmon, pork products, and vegetable proteins in addition to rabbit meal, and it was therefore not an appropriate diet trial.

The patient's obesity was best explained by chronic caloric intake in excess of his requirements due to inactivity and a reduction in lean body mass secondary to castration (1). Pathologic conditions that alter metabolic rate and predispose to obesity, such as hypothyroidism, were considered as potential risk factors. However, the age of the dog at the onset of obesity made such differential diagnoses unlikely, and the provision of energy-dense diets in excess of predicted caloric requirements during periods of concurrent glucocorticoid administration appeared most compatible with the history and clinical signs. The patient had no significant exercise and therefore no expected caloric expenditure beyond that of other sedentary pet dogs. The patient's weight was stable the 3 months prior to presentation, and it was estimated to be about 50% greater than his ideal weight of 42 kg using body conditioning scoring (each point over 5/9 consistent with an estimated 13% excess over ideal body weight) (2). The patient's caloric intake $\left(121*\text{ideal BW}_{kg}^{0.75}\right)$ therefore approximated that of laboratory dogs of similar age, a value that is generally 30% higher than that of pet dogs (1). Significant variation has been reported in most reports of maintenance energy requirements (MER) in the dog, but it was clear that a significant reduction in intake would be necessary for weight loss (3).

9.7.3 Plan

The patient's resting energy requirement $\left(\text{RER}, 70*\text{ideal BW}_{kg}^{0.75}\right)$ of about 1150 kcal was established as an initial target to achieve weight loss of 1% per week as commonly suggested (4), recognizing that large breed dogs and dogs with greater adiposity will require a greater caloric restriction relative to MER to achieve such a rate than will smaller or less overweight dogs. It was further thought that RER would be sufficient because the weight stable intake was high compared to that established for pet dogs.

The client was instructed that a home-cooked diet would be the best option for an elimination trial. Unbalanced home-cooked diets have been historically

* Dogswell Happy Hips Duck Breast, 19 kcal/treat, kcal/kg unavailable (discontinued product).

recommended during the initial food test for simplicity and to avoid confounding supplement ingredients (5,6). In this patient, such an approach would have produced severe deficiencies due to the planned caloric restriction. Consequently, a diet composed of alligator tail meat and quinoa was formulated to meet the recommended allowances (RA) for an adult dog at the patient's estimated ideal body weight (Table 9.3). A basic nutrient profile for alligator tail was located, and amino acid composition was obtained from unpublished data. Mineral and vitamin analyses were unavailable. All added supplements were evaluated for potential antigens; the only possible source was carmine (a natural colorant) in the multivitamin, but no previous patient exposure was identified. The formulated diet met or exceeded the patient's RA for most nutrients (Table 9.4), and for those nutrients less than the RA, no data was available for alligator meat and deficiencies were considered unlikely.

Dietary intake using the formulated recipe approximated 1280 kcal/day, slightly more that the established target. However, this amount was still over a one-third reduction from previous intake, and it was to be adjusted at the first recheck. Analysis of the prepared diet by a commercial laboratory was offered, but declined by the client. Recheck examinations were recommended at 3–5 week intervals, but the final monitoring was dependent on concurrent visits with the dermatologist given the distance the owner traveled. Blood work was not a required component of this patient's dietary follow-up, as the patient was young and the diet was designed for short-term feeding of a maximum of 4 to 6 weeks after resolution of the skin infections and before oral challenge. The overall nutritional prognosis was uncertain since food hypersensitivity cannot be definitively diagnosed until rechallenge with the previous diet or individual proteins (5) and because response to fatty acid supplementation in patients with other forms of allergic skin disease is unpredictable (7).

Table 9.3 Formulated novel protein diet for weight loss (average daily amounts)

Alligator tail meat	330 g
Quinoa, dry	150 g
Sunflower oil, 65% linoleic acid	2 tbsp
Flaxseed oil	2 tsp
Fish oil	1 tsp
Table salt, iodized	1/4 tsp
Lite salt	1/2 tsp
Dicalcium phosphate	1.5 tsp
Total Formula 2 (multivitamin)[a]	1 tab
Choline bitartrate, 300 mg choline/tab[b]	2 tab
L-methionine powder, 2.8 g/tsp[c]	1/4 tsp

[a] Integrative Therapeutics, Green Bay, Wisconsin.
[b] Country Life, Hauppauge, New York.
[c] Life Extension, Fort Lauderdale, Florida.

Table 9.4 Comparison of selected dietary nutrients to 2006 NRC recommended allowances (RA)

Nutrient	Units	Home-cooked diet			
		42 kg dog	Intake/day	% RA	Intake/Mcal
Energy	kcal	2145	1280	60	1000
Crude protein	g	53.6	102	191	79.8
Fat	g	29.6	59.5	201	46.5
Linoleic acid	g	6.0	22	372	18
ALA	g	0.2	5.0	2132	3.9
EPA and DHA	g	0.2	1.8	780	1.4
Calcium	g	2.1	2.1	97	1.6
Phosphorus	g	1.6	2.0	124	1.6
Vitamin A	RE	813	3000	369	2340
Cholecalciferol	μg	7.3	10	137	7.8
Vitamin E	mg	16	60	372	47
Thiamin	mg	1.2	15	1274	12
Riboflavin	mg	2.8	16	559	12
Pyridoxine	mg	0.8	25.3	3149	19.8
Niacin	mg	9.1	29.4	323	23.0
Pantothenic acid	mg	8.0	26.6	330	20.8
Cobalamin	μg	18.8	25.0	133	19.5

Exercise modification was challenging, as the sedentary habits of the dog and owner made long-distance exercise impractical. The dog's lameness on examination was mild and nonspecific so no diagnostics were recommended, although the impact of obesity on the development and severity of musculoskeletal pathology was considered (8). Limited exercise was hypothesized to have mild effects on daily energy expenditure. The client was instructed to walk the dog, increasing the time over the course of a month to a target of 30 minutes twice daily. The caloric impact of such exercise was estimated to be about 30 kcal daily above maintenance, based on a walking speed of 1.6 km/hr and an energy expenditure of 1.2 $kcal/kg^{0.75}/km$ (9). Underwater treadmill therapy was discussed, which may provide advantages in maintaining lean body mass (10), but which would only increase expenditure by 18 kcal daily more than walking on land and would be associated with additional cost (9). The owner consented to the at-home exercise protocol.

9.7.4 Follow-up

The patient lost an average of 1.6% of starting body weight per week during the first 3 weeks on the diet without observed loss of muscle mass (Table 9.5). All flavored oral medications were discontinued during that time. The patient's pruritus was reportedly improving, skin cytology was negative for cocci, and

Table 9.5 Weight history and body condition scores during the monitoring period

Week	0	3	11	14	19	23	29	35
Weight (kg)	62.7	59.6	54.8	52.8	50.4	47.9	44.9	42.3
% Loss/week[a]	—	1.6	1.0	1.2	0.9	1.2	1.0	1.0
BCS	9	9	8	8	7	7	6	5

[a] The percent loss per week is calculated as the weekly average using the weight from the previous recheck. The average rate of loss from the starting weight is 0.93% weekly.

previously initiated medical therapy was continued. No adjustments to caloric intake were made because initial rates of loss often exceed those occurring later in the weight loss period (11). The patient improved in the 4 weeks following the antibiotic course with pruritus subjectively improving from a 9 to a 2 on a 10-point scale. Unfortunately, alligator meat became unavailable, and the patient was challenged with a small amount of tilapia in an attempt to provide a different novel protein. The patient's pruritus score returned to 8–9/10 within 48 hours. The owner identified an alternate source of alligator tail and restarted the previous diet, and pruritus returned to a 4/10 in the following week.

A recheck examination at 11 weeks demonstrated an average rate of weight loss of 1% per week since the previous visit with a concurrent reduction in BCS to 8/9. The owner had been compliant with the recommended exercise protocol. Bacterial dermatitis was persistent and intradermal testing produced mild to moderate responses to dust mites, *Malassezia*, and several grasses and plants, which was inconsistent with observed clinical signs. The patient partially improved at 14 weeks, the rate of weight loss was 1% weekly, and the diet was well-tolerated. A bacterial culture revealed resistance to TMS and susceptibility to chloramphenicol, so the latter was initiated. The patient's clinical signs regressed following 8 weeks of therapy, and further patch testing for contact allergy or intradermal testing was not pursued given the patient's positive response and the ongoing suspicion for food hypersensitivity. The patient was to be challenged following a recheck examination in 6 weeks, after consulting with the dermatologist. The patient's pruritus relapsed 3 days before the recheck, and no known dietary changes were reported. The patient's BCS was 6/9 and the average weekly rate of weight loss remained 1% without any visible muscle wasting. Intradermal testing at this time was consistent with atopic dermatitis in response to aeroallergens. The dermatologist advocated continuation of the diet without challenge until the suspected atopy was managed. Immunotherapy was initiated, and a food challenge was performed 2 months later with a chicken-based over-the-counter maintenance diet, which did not lead to recurrence of clinical signs. The patient was managed on this food, and true food allergy was not suspected but rather severe intermittent atopic and bacterial dermatitis, which confounded the food trial. Nonetheless, the formulated diet and exercise modification resulted in controlled weight loss without evident muscle loss, and the dietary intake was closely monitored to ensure weight reduction to the target weight, which the patient maintained for a 4-year posttrial monitoring period.

9.7.5 Discussion

Various dietary strategies are available for the management of obesity. Generally, weight loss diets are formulated with elevated nutrient density to ensure adequacy during caloric restriction, as was the case here (4). Energy density is often reduced through the inclusion of fiber and the restriction of dietary fat. Limits on dietary fat in weight loss diets have been proposed to decrease energy density and to augment thermal energy loss, but the diet employed here was not modified in either nutrient due to the use of specific limited ingredients and in order to include elevated polyunsaturated fats. Dietary protein, however, does have a clear effect on improving weight loss. Elevated protein (>26% metabolizable energy [ME] or >75 g/Mcal) like that found in the prescribed home-prepared diet preserves lean body mass (12), and may result in increased energy expenditure and palatability (3,25). The use of exercise for weight loss appears inadequate without caloric restriction, but differences, albeit small, have been demonstrated in weight loss studies employing restriction and exercise (see Chapter 7).

The patient's juvenile-onset nonseasonal pruritus complicated management of obesity and appeared consistent with food hypersensitivity at presentation, thus necessitating further consideration before implementation of a weight loss plan. Food hypersensitivity is a type of adverse food reaction that has an unknown immunologic origin and no clear breed, sex, or age predilection (5). Both IgE-mediated immediate hypersensitivity and delayed hypersensitivity have been proposed as potential causes in dogs (5). Secretory antibodies, such as IgA, and T-cell suppression, mediated by mesenteric lymph nodes and gut associated lymphoid tissue (GALT), normally prevent aberrant response to dietary antigens (13). However, such mechanisms may fail due to mucosal barrier compromise, inadequate development of oral tolerance after birth, changes in microbial flora, or concurrent diseases (5,13). Interestingly, affected dogs predominantly display cutaneous signs, making the condition clinically indistinguishable from aeroallergen-induced atopic dermatitis. However, recent work has demonstrated altered dermal (14), but not duodenal (15), T-cell phenotypes in dogs with cutaneous food hypersensitivity. Such studies have not yet yielded useful diagnostic tests, and serum IgE levels, which were previously obtained in this patient, are both unreliable and are also elevated in dogs with atopic dermatitis (16,17). Thus, diagnosis requires a novel protein diet trial following a careful diet history (5).

No commercially available therapeutic limited ingredient diets were suitable for a novel protein trial in this patient given his extensive exposure history. Over-the-counter diets were not specifically evaluated, as some products have been shown to contain unlabeled dietary antigens (18), and it was improbable that such diets would be suitable for weight loss. Hydrolyzed diets were considered. However, food hypersensitivity can occur with low molecular weight hydrolysates if the complete protein is allergenic in a particular patient (19). Such diets are also low in protein (16.5%–18% ME, or 47–52 g/Mcal), presumably due to processing costs and to guard against the unlikely event there is a dose-dependent response to a dietary allergen (5). As a result, no available diets provided the necessary features of a novel high-protein diet formulated for weight loss.

The diet included specific modifications of dietary polyunsaturated fatty acids (PUFAs). Modifications of PUFAs have been extensively mentioned in the management of human and canine atopic disease, generally arising from environmental rather than food allergens (7). However, such manipulations may be of benefit in food hypersensitivity and a portion of patients will display sensitivity to both food and aeroallergens (5,20). Historically, the focus has been on increasing omega-3 fatty acids (7), but linoleic acid is critical to stabilize the stratum corneum barrier and the wisdom of n-6 PUFA restriction in human atopy is being questioned (21). As a result, the diet was formulated with elevated amounts of both n-3 and n-6 PUFAs. No consistent dose recommendations have been reported (22,23), so the inclusions were guided by recommended allowances of essential fatty acids (1).

Diet and exercise likely both contributed to weight loss in this patient. The complex symptoms and clinical picture warranted the use of a custom-tailored nutritional strategy, which was successful, in partnership with a compliant owner, in achieving the goals for the patient. Extended monitoring of weight loss patients is necessary as rebound weight gain is common (24).

KEY LEARNING ISSUES

1. The target rate of weight loss for most dogs is between 0.5% and 2% weekly, and rates of weight loss in the first few weeks may be higher.
2. The management of obesity with other nutritionally responsive conditions may require customization of an animal's diet plan.
3. Home-prepared diets can be used for weight loss with careful planning and inclusion of some of the dietary factors known to increase the probability of weight loss success such as high protein content. Consultation with a board certified veterinary nutritionist is recommended.

REFERENCES

1. National Research Council (NRC) Ad Hoc Committee on Dog and Cat. *Nutrient Requirements of Dogs and Cats*. Washington DC: National Academies Press; 2006.
2. German AJ, Holden SL, Bissot T et al. Use of starting condition score to estimate changes in body weight and composition during weight loss in obese dogs. *Research in Veterinary Science* 2009;87(2):249–254.
3. Diez M, Nguyen P, Jeusette I et al. Weight loss in obese dogs: Evaluation of a high protein, low-carbohydrate diet. *The Journal of Nutrition* 2002;132(6):1685S–1687S.
4. Brooks D, Churchill J, Fein K et al. 2014 AAHA weight management guidelines for dogs and cats. *Journal of the American Animal Hospital Association* 2014;50:1–11.

5. Verlinden A, Hesta M, Millet S et al. Food allergy in dogs and cats: A review. *Critical Reviews in Food Science and Nutrition* 2006;46(3):259–273.

6. Roudebush P, Cowell CS. Results of a hypoallergenic diet survey of veterinarians in North America with a nutritional evaluation of homemade diet prescriptions. *Veterinary Dermatology* 1992;3(1):23–28.

7. Mueller RS, Fieseler KV, Fettman MJ et al. Effect of omega-3 fatty acids on canine atopic dermatitis. *Journal of Small Animal Practice* 2004;45(6):293–297.

8. Marshall W, Hazelwinkel H, Mullen D et al. The effect of weight loss on lameness in obese dogs with osteoarthritis. *Veterinary Research Communications* 2010;34(3):241–253.

9. Shmalberg J, Scott KC, Williams JM, Hill RC. Energy expenditure of dogs exercising on an underwater treadmill compared to that on a dry treadmill. *13th Annual AAVN Clinical Nutrition and Research Symposium,* Seattle, Washington; 2013.

10. Vitger AD, Stallknecht BM, Nielsen DH, Bjornvad CR. Integration of a physical training program in a weight loss plan for overweight pet dogs. *Journal of American Veterinary Medical Association* 2016;248(2):174–182.

11. Fritsch DA, Ahle NW, Jewell DE et al. A high-fiber food improves weight loss compared to a high-protein, high-fat food in pet dogs in a home setting. *The Journal of Applied Research in Veterinary Medicine* 2010;8(3):138–145.

12. Hannah SS, Laflamme DP. Increased dietary protein spares lean body mass during weight loss in dogs (ACVIM abstract). *Journal of Veterinary Internal Medicine* 1998;12:224.

13. Brandtzaeg P. Food allergy: Separating the science from the mythology. *Nature Reviews Gastroenterology and Hepatology* 2010;7:380–400.

14. Veenhof EZ, Knol EF, Schlotter YM et al. Characterisation of T cell phenotypes, cytokines and transcription factors in the skin of dogs with cutaneous adverse food reactions. *The Veterinary Journal* 2011;187(3):320–324.

15. Veenhof EZ, Rutten VP, van Noort R et al. Evaluation of T-cell activation in the duodenum of dogs with cutaneous food hypersensitivity. *American Journal of Veterinary Research* 2010;71(4):441–446.

16. Jackson HA, Jackson MW, Coblentz L et al. Evaluation of the clinical and allergen specific serum immunoglobulin E responses to oral challenge with cornstarch, corn, soy and a soy hydrolysate diet in dogs with spontaneous food allergy. *Veterinary Dermatology* 2003;14(4):181–187.

17. Foster AP, Knowles TG, Moore AH et al. Serum IgE and IgG responses to food antigens in normal and atopic dogs, and dogs with gastrointestinal disease. *Veterinary Immunology and Immunopathology* 2003;92(3–4):113–124.

18. Raditic DM, Remillard RL, Tater KC. ELISA testing for common food antigens in four dry dog foods used in dietary elimination trials. *Journal of Animal Physiology and Animal Nutrition* 2011;95(1):90–97.

19. Cave NJ. Hydrolyzed protein diets for dogs and cats. *Veterinary Clinics of North America: Small Animal Practice* 2006;36(6):1251–1268.
20. Nesbitt GH, Freeman LM, Hannah SS. Effect of n-3 fatty acid ratio and dose on clinical manifestations, plasma fatty acids and inflammatory mediators in dogs with pruritus. *Veterinary Dermatology* 2003;14(2):67–74.
21. Sala-Vila A, Miles EA, Calder PC. Fatty acid composition abnormalities in atopic disease: Evidence explored and role in the disease process examined. *Clinical & Experimental Allergy* 2008;38(9):1432–1450.
22. Bauer JE. Therapeutic use of fish oils in companion animals. *Journal of the American Veterinary Medical Association* 2011;239(11):1441–1451.
23. Lenox CE. Timely topics in nutrition: An overview of fatty acids in companion animal medicine. *Journal of the American Veterinary Medical Association* 2015;246(11):1198–1202.
24. Laflamme DP, Kuhlman G. The effect of weight loss regimen on subsequent weight maintenance in dogs. *Nutrition Research* 1995;15(7): 1019–1028.
25. Toll PW, Yamka RM, Schoenherr WD et al. *Obesity.* In Hand MS, Thatcher CD, Remillard RL et al. (eds.) Small Animal Clinical Nutrition. Topeka, Kansas: Mark Morris Institute, 2010;502–542.

9.8 CASE 8: VETERINARY NURSE INVOLVEMENT WITH WEIGHT LOSS PLANS

ASHLEY COX

9.8.1 Patient history

A 7-year-old, female, spayed, obese Pembroke Welsh corgi presented to a veterinary teaching hospital's clinical nutrition service for a weight loss plan. Sugar was newly adopted from a corgi rescue with minimally available medical history. The new owner was very committed to helping Sugar achieve weight loss.

9.8.2 Diet history

Preceding the initial appointment, Sugar's owner had completed a diet, activity and household history form (DAHHF) that was e-mailed from the receptionists at the time of scheduling the appointment. The owner was asked to e-mail the completed form or bring it in at the time of the appointment. Upon presentation, the veterinary nurse weighed Sugar and reviewed the diet history. Prior to adoption, Sugar was consuming 3/4 cup twice daily of two dry diets mixed in equal proportions, providing an estimated 577 kcal per day. Since adoption, approximately 2 months prior, the owner had reduced the diet to 3/8 cup twice daily, 1 cup of green beans per day as treats, and one joint health supplement soft chew. During this 2-month period, her estimated daily intake was 299 kcal from diet (74% of daily kcal), 47 kcal from treats, and an estimated 58 kcal from supplements (26% of daily kcal), totaling 394 kcal per day. The owner was not sure, but thought Sugar may have lost some weight during this time.

9.8.3 Patient assessment

At initial presentation, Sugar's physical exam was unremarkable except for an obese body condition. The veterinarian and veterinary nurse palpated Sugar and estimated a body condition score (BCS) of 9/9 with an estimated 50%–55% body fat, normal muscle conditioning with a weight of 18.4 kilograms (40.4 lb). Baseline complete blood count (CBC), chemistry, total thyroxine (T4), and urinalysis were unremarkable. At this time, photos were taken of Sugar as she was standing, being sure to include a view from above, side (Figure 9.6a) and back. These photos were added to Sugar's medical record. After the owner signed a photo release form, the photos were added to the weight loss participant board displayed in the client waiting area.

9.8.4 Plan

Based upon an estimated 52.5% body fat, and following the 2014 AAHA weight management guidelines for dogs and cats, Sugar's estimated ideal body weight (BW) was calculated (1).

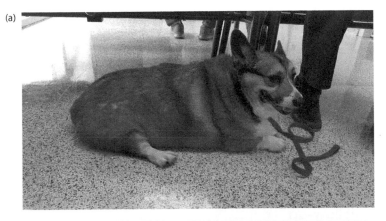

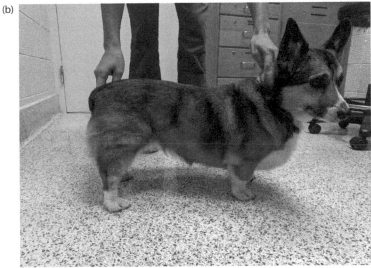

Figure 9.6 **(a)** Before (week 0) and **(b)** after (week 52) side profile photos.

Calculation of ideal BW:

$$18.4\,\text{kg} \times (100\% - 52.5\%)/80\% = 10.9\,\text{kg}\;(24.0\,\text{lb})$$

Resting energy requirement (RER) was estimated to be 420 kcal per day (1). Calculation of resting energy requirement (RER):

$$\text{RER} = 70 \times (\text{ideal BW}_{kg})^{0.75} = 70 \times 10.9^{0.75} = 420\,\text{kcal/day}$$

Calculation of daily energy allocation for weight loss:

$$= 1.0 \times 420 = 420\,\text{kcal/day}$$
$$= 0.8 \times 420 = 336\,\text{kcal/day}$$

It was recommended to feed 360 kcal from a therapeutic weight loss diet with an additional 40 kcal from treats and supplements, totaling 400 kcal per day. At the time of the initial appointment, owners have the option to purchase a "weight loss package" to include the initial appointment and 12 monthly weight rechecks with the veterinary nurse at a discounted package price or paying for each individual nurse recheck appointment. Sugar's owner purchased the weight loss package and scheduled for a 4-week nurse recheck appointment. Before being discharged the owner was encouraged to participate within the private Facebook* page for all weight loss program participants and join monthly support meetings offered at the clinic. Sugar was provided with a "jump-start" package to inspire adherence throughout the weight loss venture.

9.8.5 Follow-up

Due to preemptively scheduling her recheck date and a reminder phone call from a client service representative, Sugar returned for her first weight recheck in 6 weeks. Her body weight at this time was 16.7 kg (36.7 lb) with a weight loss of 1.7 kg (3.7 lb) or 9.2% of her body weight. She was reported to be eating the new diet well and her caloric intake was reviewed to ensure adherence to the weight loss program. She was still receiving green beans as treats, about 2/3 cup daily with 1 tablespoon of canned pumpkin (31.6 kcal from treats) and half of a joint health supplement soft chew (12 kcal from supplements). The daily meals and treats totaled an estimated 404 calories per day with 89% from the diet and 11% from treats and supplements. Although calories from treats marginally exceeded the recommended 10%, Sugar was losing at a rate of 1.5% of her body weight per week (Box 9.1) and the feeding plan was maintained. Sugar returned approximately every 4 weeks for 7 months with an appropriate rate of weight loss.

BOX 9.1: Calculating rate of weight loss per week

$$\text{Total rate of weight loss} = \frac{(\text{Previous weight} - \text{Current weight})}{\text{Previous weight}} \times 100$$

$$\text{Sugar's total rate of weight loss} = [(18.4 \text{ kgs} - 16.7 \text{ kgs})/18.4 \text{ kgs}] \times 100 = 9.2\%$$

$$\text{Weekly rate of weight loss} = \frac{\text{Total rate of weight loss}}{\#\text{Weeks since previous weight}}$$

$$\text{Sugar's weekly rate of weight loss} = 9.2\%/6 \text{ weeks} = 1.5\%$$

---

* Facebook, Inc., Menlo Park, California.

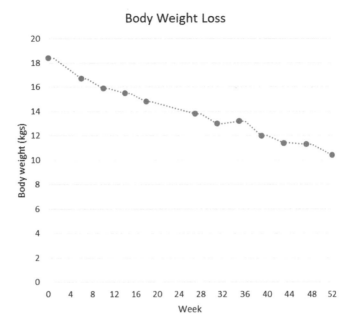

Figure 9.7 Body weight loss history over 12 months.

At her 7-month recheck, Sugar's body weight plateaued. A review of her caloric intake revealed that the owner had not altered any of the dietary components from the amounts last reported. It was recommended to start weighing the dry food in grams on a kitchen scale to improve precision when feeding (2). Treat dispensing toys and automatic feeders were discussed with the owner as options to remove the association of the owner to meal feedings. Following the switch to gram measurements, feeding at 80% of RER (decrease of 68 kcal) within a treat dispensing toy, and attending monthly support meetings and nurse recheck appointments, Sugar was able to reach her ideal weight of 10.4 kg (23 lb) one year from her initial weight loss appointment (Figure 9.7). Repeat photos were taken as described earlier and added to her medical chart (Figure 9.6b). These photos were then printed onto a certificate and given to Sugar's owner, along with a new collar. Overall, Sugar lost 7.9 kg (17.4 lb) during her weight loss program. To encourage weight maintenance, her caloric intake was increased by 5% (17 calorie increase, 353 calories per day) using her current therapeutic weight loss diet. A weight recheck was scheduled for one month to continue to monitor her weight maintenance phase and to adjust her caloric intake, if needed.

9.8.6 Discussion

Veterinary nurses can be an integral part of successful weight loss programs in client-owned pets. Being able to review and collect an accurate diet history, including the main diet, treats, foods used for medication administration, and supplements, will establish a strong foundation for the veterinarian to make appropriate dietary recommendations. Remaining an active part of the pet's weight loss and engaging the owner(s) as much as possible can encourage adherence and relieve some of the obstacles and/or stress that comes with pet weight loss programs. Creating a board within the waiting area that has photos of all participating pets with their side profile, monthly weights, and ultimate weight loss goals may help motivate clients, providing friendly competition or even the comfort of knowing that their pet is not the only one to plateau during weight loss. The private Facebook page or other social media sites for weight loss program participants provides a social environment for owners to confide and encourage one another. It may also be used as a tool for the veterinary team to educate clients about obesity.

Veterinary nurses have the opportunity to provide empathy and management strategies when owners feel defeated and struggle with common roadblocks associated with weight loss. Commonly, this includes exhausting begging behaviors. There are numerous treat dispensing toys offering the flexibility and complexity necessary to be used for meal feedings. The treat toys used for meals can increase the time it takes for total food consumption potentially providing enrichment, satiety, and increases in activity. If the owner finds that the pet becomes frustrated with treat dispensing toys or is not food motivated enough to use them, feeding the pet within a room that is minimally used may decrease owner-directed begging behavior. For example, if the patient is currently fed in the kitchen and the owner frequently goes into the kitchen, the pet may think that every entry into the kitchen has the potential to result in the provision of a treat or other food item. Instead, feed in a room that is rarely visited, such as the guest bathroom or bedroom. Ideally, removing the owner completely from feeding and relying on an automatic feeding device may help to encourage begging toward the inanimate feeder instead of the owner.

Scheduling the recheck nurse appointment before the owner leaves their current appointment defines a commitment upon the owner. Reminder communications through the support staff as the appointment gets closer ensures adherence and facilitates rescheduling if needed. To help inspire and motivate the clients, "jump-start" packages may be given at their first visit. Suggested items to include in these packages are a sample of the therapeutic diet, measuring cup, can lid, a new leash, and reading material (e.g., weight loss success stories, flyer for monthly support meetings, understanding body condition scoring, and medical consequences of obesity). The monthly support meetings may include various topics ranging from appropriate activities for overweight pets, owner success stories, general nutrition question-and-answer sessions, or group pet swims at an indoor rehabilitation pool.

Weight loss programs have the potential to positively impact the pet, owner(s), and the veterinary clinic when managed appropriately. A veterinary nurse trained on how to educate clients, obtain a detailed diet history, manage weight loss, discuss obstacles, and troubleshoot with the owner can improve pet weight loss success. The veterinary nurse should assist the veterinarian with the initial consultation, but once trained can manage the weight loss rechecks with veterinary oversight. Once the pet has reached their estimated ideal/target body weight, the veterinarian and veterinary nurse should recheck and finalize the long-term weight maintenance plan. Overall, weight loss appointments require dedication and commitment from everyone involved. Veterinary nurses are an excellent resource when working with veterinarians to successfully lead and support owners and their pets through all the challenging aspects of weight loss.

KEY LEARNING POINTS

1. Veterinary nurses should be trained and comfortable with reviewing and collecting an accurate and complete diet history. Accuracy in the diet history can influence the caloric estimates used in determining the weight loss plan. Inaccuracies can create undesirable weight gain or loss when initiating the plan.
2. A pet's weight loss commonly plateaus! So, effectively guiding and motivating owners through times of hardship by being creative with food administration and encouraging interaction through group meetings and social media can encourage continued participation.
3. All things in moderation; treats can be a way for owners to feel connected with their pet and do not need to be excluded from the diet plan to obtain successful weight loss. Discuss with owners the importance of a caloric allotment for treats in maintaining the overall balance of the therapeutic diet and overall weight loss success.
4. It is important to find the nonnegotiables. In reviewing the diet history, identify habitual treats. For example, the owner reads a book at night before bed and they must provide their pet with a treat to relax while they read. This is important to the owner and their pet, therefore working to provide a treat that fits within the calorie allotment can influence the overall compliance to the weight loss plan.
5. Supplements may provide calories. Be sure to account for calories coming from supplements as part of the treat allotment.

REFERENCES

1. Brooks D, Churchill J, Fein K et al. 2014 AAHA weight management guidelines for dogs and cats. *Journal of the American Animal Hospital Association* 2014;50:1–11.
2. German AJ, Holden SL, Mason SL et al. Imprecision when using measuring cups to weigh out extruded dry kibbled food. *Journal of Animal Physiology and Animal Nutrition* 2011;95:368–373. https://www.ncbi.nlm.nih.gov/pubmed/21039926

Index

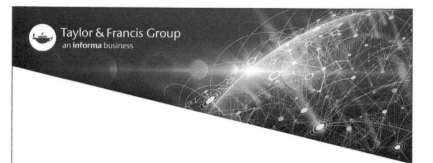